The Book of Yoga Self-Practice

20 tools to help you create and sustain
a fulfilling independent yoga practice

About the Author

Rebecca Anderton-Davies, also known as RAD and Somewhat RAD, is a yoga practitioner and teacher, online community founder, author, investment banker, wife and mother.

Yoga came into her life when she was in her late twenties and was hit by a truck cycling to work. Some 6 months later she was struggling with her injuries and on the advice of a physiotherapist turned to yoga. Slowly and with many challenges along the way, she went from being unable to touch her toes to a qualified yoga teacher.

At the same time she was progressing in her career as an investment banker, and becoming a mother to an energetic son.

Rebecca's message, which she shares with her Instagram community (@somewhat_rad), centres on developing a bespoke, creative, independent yoga practice which can fit in with even the busiest of lives.

Rebecca started teaching her yoga self-practice workshops in 2017 and founded the Yoga Self-Practice community in 2018 to be a place where real people practicing real yoga could see themselves represented online. It has now grown to overtake her personal account and inspired *The Book of Yoga Self-Practice*, her tool to enable readers to develop and maintain their very own yoga self-practice. Read more about Rebecca's story on page 312.

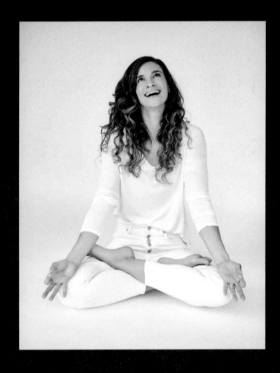

The Book of Yoga Self-Practice

20 tools to help you create and sustain a fulfilling independent yoga practice

Rebecca Anderton-Davies

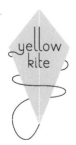

First published in Great Britain in 2020
by Yellow Kite
An imprint of Hodder & Stoughton
An Hachette UK company

2

Text © RAD Innovations Ltd 2020
Illustrations © RAD Innovations Ltd 2020
Illustrations by Chiara Pennella 2020
Design by Simon Anderton 2020
Author image © Elisabeth Hoff 2020: page 2

The information given in this book
should not be treated as a substitute for
professional medical advice; always consult
a medical practitioner. Any use of information
in this book is at the reader's discretion and
risk. Neither the author nor the publisher
can be held responsible for any loss, claim
or damage arising out of the use, or misuse,
of the suggestions made, the failure to
take medical advice or for any material on
third-party websites.

A CIP catalogue record for this title is available
from the British Library

Trade paperback ISBN 978 1 529 34946 7
eBook ISBN 978 1 529 34947 4

Colour origination by Altaimage
Printed and bound in Italy by Lego S.p.A

Hodder & Stoughton policy is to use papers
that are natural, renewable and recyclable
products and made from wood grown
in sustainable forests. The logging and
manufacturing processes are expected to
conform to the environmental regulations
of the country of origin.

Yellow Kite
Hodder & Stoughton Ltd
Carmelite House
50 Victoria Embankment
London EC4Y 0DZ

www.yellowkite.co.uk
www.hodder.co.uk

To Nick and to Quinn.
My boys.
My loves.

This book was lovingly (and patiently!)
designed by Simon Anderton
www.makeideasmatter.xyz
@agentbright777

Contents

I'm
Rebecca

A.K.A RAD

A.K.A @somewhat_rad

I'm Rebecca, the founder of Yoga Self-Practice.

Yoga Self-Practice is a community dedicated to providing the TOOLS you need to CREATE and to SUSTAIN a fulfilling independent yoga practice.

My priority is getting you tools that you can use in and around your practice. This comes over and above teaching specific yoga poses or precise flows. Because the power of yoga as a system – of movement, of mindfulness, and of spirituality – lies in its diversity and flexibility. And NOTHING is more diverse or flexible or ultimately bespoke to you and your body and your life than a self-practice.

This book contains all the tools you need to start, develop and improve your yoga self-practice.

It is the in-depth resource I wish I had had with me when I started out on my own self-practice journey.

You can read about how that journey began for me at the end of this book, and there are more resources to help you at www.yoga-self-practice.com. But for now, read on, and remember: if you keep showing up for yoga, it will keep showing up for you.

Happy self-practicing

Introduction

This book
will show
you how to
**take the next
step** in your
**journey of yoga
self-practice.**

I say **next** very deliberately.

The first step was the moment you decided you wanted to start, or further develop, your independent yoga practice.

You can be led by a teacher in a class. You can be persuaded by a friend to do a yoga challenge on Instagram. You can half-heartedly follow a video online. But no one can flip the switch for you to start a yoga self-practice. Or force you onto your mat as you work to improve it.

It took your willpower, your decision making, and your commitment both to your *practice* and to *yourself* to do that. These qualities – willpower, decision making and commitment – will strengthen and grow as you build your yoga self-practice and will be what sustains it.

Most of us think of the physical practice of the postures when we talk about 'yoga', and the physical benefits will often be what brings us to the mat, at least initially. But you are most likely here because you ALSO want the mental, emotional and perhaps even spiritual benefits that come with a regular and consistent practice.

I point all of this out because I want you to see that you are already flexing the mental muscles needed for self-practice. These mental muscles will lead to changes in the physical ones, which in turn will further develop your mental strength. And on and on it will go.

This isn't an impossible task that you will never master. **You are already doing it.**

Yoga stills the mind's fluctuations

योगश्चत्तिवृत्तनिरोधः ॥२॥
yogaś citta-vṛtti-nirodhaḥ

yoga

SUTRAS 1.2

the Asana

This book focuses on the physical element of yoga practice.

I focus on **the asana** because the physical practice is how most people find themselves discovering the wonderful system that is yoga.

According to the Yoga Sūtras
of Patañjali – a collection of 196
observations on the theory and
practice of yoga, compiled around
the year AD400 by the
renowned Indian sage –

Asana is just one of the eight limbs of the practice that the term 'yoga' encompasses.

eight limbs of yoga

YAMA
Restraints, moral disciplines or moral vows

NIYAMA
Positive duties or observances

ASANA
Physical postures

PRANAYAMA
Breathing techniques

PRATYAHARA
Withdrawal of the senses

DHARANA
Focused concentration

DHYANA
Meditative absorption

SAMADHI
Bliss or enlightenment

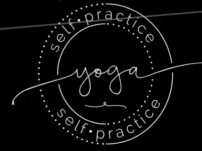

self·practice
yoga
self·practice

So why asana?
No one says
it better than
one of the first
teachers to
bring yoga
to the West,
B.K.S. Iyengar:

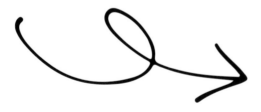

"

Asana practice brings mind and body into harmony for this task. Your mind is always ahead of your body. You mind moves into the future, the body the past, but the self is in the present. The coordination between them that we learn in asana will enable us to turn the shape of our visions into the substance of our lives …

… In relation to the body, this means that we are not our body in any permanent sense, but for all practical purposes, we are our bodies, because they are the vehicle through which we perceive and can discover our immortality.

This is why yoga begins with the body.

So, we start with our bodies. We start with the physical practice. And then we can begin to access everything else that yoga offers.

Physical practice is the gateway to the other limbs of yoga, particularly for people (like us!) who live increasingly digital lives.

With days spent moving words, ideas, and money electronically around the world, and evenings spent tending to virtual relationships through social media, it can be easy to lose focus on that which is tangible and concrete.

The physical practice of asana is a shock, often an incredibly difficult one, that brings us back to the vessel we rely on, yet often ignore, to achieve everything else.

What might look a little strange in a book focused on the physical practice of yoga is that there are no set instructions here on how to do a single posture. **Zero. Zilch. Nada.**

Nothing about where to place a foot or a hand, or which muscles to engage, or where to take the focus of your eyes.

This may seem even stranger given that the biggest hurdle to starting a yoga self-practice for many people is fear of hurting themselves without being under the watchful eye of a skilled teacher or the fear of doing it 'wrong'.

Surely any book on yoga practice, especially a yoga SELF-practice, needs to have instructions on how to do a Downward Facing Dog?!

This book focuses on the (physical) PRACTICE of yoga. Everything here is geared towards you maximising the opportunities to practice. The content of that practice, as long as you are not compromising your long-term health, is not particularly important.

Let me explain...

Right & Wrong in a Physical Yoga Practice

Is there a 'right' way to do a yoga pose?

Namaskars, or movements and mantras as rituals to be offered at sunrise and sunset, were first described in the *Rig Veda*, the oldest collection of sacred Hindu scriptures, which is over 3,500 years old.

However, it is broadly agreed that the physical asana practice that we would recognise today developed in India between 1920 and 1940. This development was led by Jagannath G. Gune and then his student Tirumalai Krishnamacharya, who in turn taught Sri K. Pattabhi Jois and B.K.S. Iyengar. The two men who 'brought yoga to the West' in the 1960s.

Fascinatingly, even though these two men (Jois and Iyengar) were taught by the same teacher, they went on to found two very different schools of yoga. The slower practice of Iyengar; where the emphasis is on transforming the pose to fit the person with the use of a multitude of props. Versus the faster paced and methodical practice of Ashtanga; where yogis follow a strict set of prescribed poses and are only allowed to progress onto the next one once their teacher is happy they have mastered the current one.

Even at the start, the experts had different takes on what the 'right' way of doing things was.

Scroll forward nearly a century, and many more styles of yoga have developed. In turn, many Yoga Teaching Training (YTT) courses have been established.

This new industry is entirely self-regulated. Private non-profits such as the Yoga Alliance, based in the US, have taken the lead in setting their own standards of proficiency for both yoga schools and the certified 'yoga teachers' they produce – settling on 200 hours (around four weeks of full-time study) as a basic level, and 500 hours for an advanced level.

Other schools of yoga have their own rules. Bikram yoga requires teachers to take a nine-week course. Iyengar teachers meanwhile must pass the toughest training: they are required to have studied the practice for a minimum of two years, before they then undertake two years of training and pass two exams in order to call themselves an official Iyengar Yoga teacher. Unsurprisingly, the content of all of these courses varies hugely.

This multitude of yoga experts don't agree on the best way of teaching teachers and they don't agree on the best way of executing a Downward Facing Dog.

The 'right' way to do a yoga pose depends on who you ask.

Won't I be safer practicing with a teacher?

A particular teacher's instruction may suit most bodies, but your body could be different. Or you may find it difficult to translate their instructions in to action.

Or their attention may be with one of the other 20, or 30, or 40 students in front of them.

Many teachers will have taken many teacher training courses, and practiced and taught thousands of hours of yoga. They may have combined all of this with evidence-based trainings requiring degree-level study, such as physiotherapy. But many teachers will have just completed the minimum 200 hours of training over a matter of a few weeks (myself included!). So which teacher are you practicing with?

Even in a class, you are taking a risk by solely relying on a teacher to 'protect' you from doing a pose in a way that leads to injuries. The truth is that, even with a teacher present, risks remain. No one is in your body apart from you.

Amazing teachers have the power to transform your yoga practice. And as you will see, this book encourages you again and again to go out and learn from them. But they do not – they CANNOT – have all the answers.

But surely there is a 'wrong' way to do a pose?

Over the past few decades, there have been numerous studies published on the physical benefits and potential injury risks associated with yoga practice.

One of the most accessible ways to understand the science is to read William J. Broad's book *The Science of Yoga*, which takes you on an incredibly well researched tour of what this research says.

The most terrifying pieces of research he highlights found that certain postures (such as plow and shoulderstand), when badly executed, can cause strokes. As a result, Broad has removed these poses from his own practice. He also explains how some teachers who have taken on this evidence have modified their teaching of these postures.

Indeed, most long-term yoga practitioners will have a story to tell about how they pushed themselves too hard, or did a pose badly, or a teacher adjusted them poorly, and they hurt themselves.

So yes, you can absolutely injure yourself doing yoga. And if you injure yourself, either in a moment or over long-term misuse of your body, then you are doing something 'wrong'.

Having a basic knowledge of how to protect yourself from injury is absolutely essential when conducting ANY physical activity. This is why there is an entire section of this book dedicated to helping you decide whether you have a solid enough foundation to start a yoga self-practice. Beyond that, many of the tools laid out here are specifically to encourage you to learn both about your body and the practice.

However, just because you can hurt yourself doing something wrong, it doesn't mean there is a right way of doing it. There are safer ways, and less safe ways for different bodies, with different levels of strength and flexibility and history of movement; what is safe for your body may not be safe for my body.

The only 'right' way is what is right for you and **your specific purpose** in **that specific moment** of **that specific practice**.

A self-practice forces you to take responsibility working out what all those things are. Which can be scary!

Knowing there is no 'right' answer is hard. Knowing that you will need to go out and seek a variety of different opinions and then find the one which is the 'most' right FOR YOU can feel like a daunting task.

Accepting that the consequences of what you choose to do and how you choose to do it are all on you can be overwhelming.

However, by acknowledging, accepting and ultimately embracing this responsibility, I believe you start to learn more, progress faster, and experience more deeply the many and varied benefits that yoga brings.

You will learn more about your own body because you are paying so much more attention to it as it moves. You will progress faster with tuning into the tricks your mind can play on you because you are giving yourself the space to listen.

After all, we don't practice yoga asana to get better at yoga asana. We practice yoga asana to get better at **living**.

Don't get too hung up on doing the poses perfectly, always prioritise your safety and your long-term health, and you will be doing it as 'right' as it is possible to be.

Why Vinyasa?

This book centres around the Vinyasa style of yoga. Vinyasa yoga is a style which focuses on linking poses together in a flowing fashion.

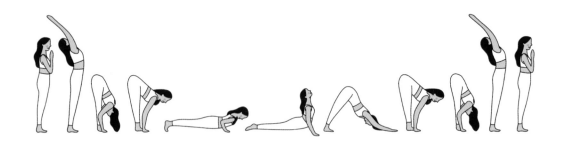

Its true beauty is that this can be done in a multitude of ways: fast or slow, holding postures or not, seated or standing. It can be practiced with or without music, in a hot room or with a big cuddly jumper on, for 5 minutes or 500 minutes. Anything and everything goes in Vinyasa.

A Vinyasa yoga practice encourages you to adapt your practice to suit your needs – be they physical, mental or spiritual – EVERY SINGLE TIME you practice.

Which, in my view, is exactly what a yoga practice should be about. Especially a self-practice.

However, if reading this book makes you realise a Vinyasa self-practice isn't for you, THAT'S OK! Maybe you already know you prefer a different style of yoga. You are more than welcome to use the tools here to help with your Yin self-practice or take the advice into your Hatha self-practice.

You may decide that you actually crave the structure of the fixed Ashtanga sequence. Or realise that carving out the time to go to a studio is the best option for you, or that those online classes you take really are working. If so, there are still tools here which you can use to help you on that path, especially in Parts 4 and 5.

Everything here is about helping you work out what works FOR YOU. Take what does, leave what doesn't, and congratulate yourself for the progress that indicates you've made.

The **tools** you need to **create** & to **sustain** a fulfilling **yoga** self-practice

This book contains 20 tools to inspire and support you to develop your own yoga self-practice.

These are designed to help you find a yoga self-practice that works for you: independent and totally bespoke.

That this book is over 300 pages may make it seem that a yoga self-practice requires a huge amount of work. This is absolutely not the case.

In fact, the less you have to plan and prepare, the more you are going to practice.

We are all busy, and we all have limited stores of energy and willpower. Use this energy to practice and not on planning your practice.

There are people who get paid cold hard cash to design, remember, and stick to perfectly structured sequences: YOGA TEACHERS! Sadly, I haven't figured out a way to get you paid in a similar way for a similar amount of effort in your self-practice.

So how about we just reduce the effort at the planning stage and instead save it for when you are on your mat?!

The quantity of planning and preparation that is just enough is going to vary wildly from day to day. Some days you might want it to be a decent amount. This book will take you through techniques you can use when you stumble into one of those days. In Part 8 (page 280) I'll be introducing you to blank templates that you can use again and again if this method works for you. You can also head to www.yoga-self-practice.com to download these so you can print or keep them handy on all your digital devices.

Other days, just enough planning and preparation will be precisely ZERO planning and preparation. Which is why many of the tools here will give you the inspiration for an entire practice without any at all.

This book provides prompts, options, ideas, suggestions. Use one, use them all, mix and match. Use one on Monday, seven on Tuesday. Consider them and discard them, for today's practice, for all future practices. It is totally up to you.

With these 20 tools, the bar for you to actually practice will hopefully be as low as possible, while your practice itself will be as fulfilling and enjoyable as possible. **Because then, you will keep coming back to it again, and again, and again.**

Starting or developing a yoga self-practice can feel overwhelming. I am simply going to ask you to not let it be.

Read this quote
from Michael A. Singer
in his book *The Untethered Soul*

"

If you mistreat an animal, it becomes afraid.
That is what has happened to your psyche.
You have mistreated it by giving it a responsibility
that is incomprehensible. Just stop for a moment
and see what you have given your mind to do.

You said to your mind, 'I want everyone to like me.
I don't want anyone to speak badly of me.
I want everything I say and do to be acceptable to
pleasing to everyone. I don't want anyone to hurt
me. I don't want anything to happen that I don't like.
And I want everything to happen that I do like.'

Then you said, 'Now, mind, figure out to make every
one of these things a reality, even if you have to think
about it all day and night.' And of course, your mind
said, 'I'm on the job. I will work on it constantly.'

"

Can you imagine trying to do that?

Please, please, please do not make your yoga self-practice an additional incomprehensible responsibility to your psyche's already long list!

Trust that you are a smart, complex and wonderful creature designed to continuously learn, with a body that is designed to be used.

Just trust. And try.
And trust and try again
- you've got this

How to Use This Book

This book is written so you can progress through it naturally, front to back, building the foundation and development of your self-practice in a way that flows as sequentially as possible. Many of the tools work best when used together, so these connections are flagged as well.

However, every part has also been written to answer a key question you might have about your self-practice.

So please feel free to jump straight to where your biggest hurdle lies:

Part 2

Am I ready for a self-practice?

Part 3

How do I know what to practice?

How do I flow by myself?

How do I structure an entire practice?

Part 4

Why is self-practice important for me?

How do I make a self-practice actually happen?

Part 5

How do I ensure progression while self-practicing?

Part 6

Troubleshooting more specific FAQs

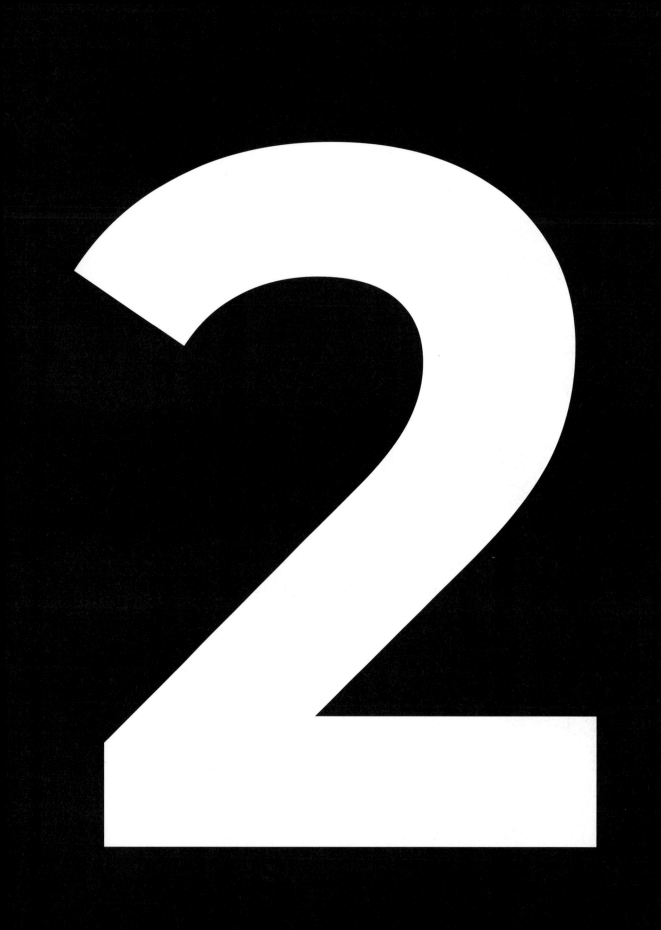

Getting Ready
for Your Mat

"

Yoga is the journey of the self,
through the self, to the self

The *Bhagavad Gita*

"

The
WHO

Am I Ready for a Self-Practice?

Yoga, including self-practice, is for everyone. Every body type, age, sex, level of fitness, flexibility, and prior experience of sport or movement.

However, a self-practice does differ to a led-practice. Whether you are following the lead of a teacher in a class, or from a YouTube video, or perhaps a reference book, this book is ideally aimed at people who already have a foundational level of practice but have never self-practiced before.

I am **brand new to yoga**

Let me be very honest with you. If you are a total beginner to yoga this guide may not be the best place to start. Or at least not the ONLY resource you need to start. As you will see, this book doesn't contain lots of instruction on how to do different poses or sequences.

When you are alone on your mat, you do need a solid enough foundation to build on: a level of knowledge of what the postures are, how to do them safely for your body, and in a way that works for whatever goals you have for your practice. Not all postures, and not even everything there is to know about the ones you do know, but enough to get started. There is an entire section on the next page to help you work out how to get started if you need some help: I know how confusing the world of yoga can be at this stage, believe me!

Use this book alongside whatever path you decide to tread to build that foundation. If you begin your yoga journey with your goal being to have an independent self-practice – be that in a class or by following videos or reading books – I almost guarantee that you will learn MORE and you will learn FASTER because you will not fall so easily into the trap of waiting for an instruction to come. You will be thinking, even sub-consciously, about how you would do this pose or that sequence or this transition when you are by yourself. Amazingly, even many 'more experienced' yogis don't do this. Really.

So, do please read on and see what this self-practice malarkey is all about.

I'm think I'm **ready to start my self-practice**

Starting a self-practice can seem like a catch-22 situation. You want to get 'good' enough to start. But how are you going to get 'good' enough without giving it a go, especially if you are focused on a self-practice because it fits better into your life than in-studio classes.

It does not have to be like this! But you do need a foundational level of practice.

Why? At the risk of pointing out the obvious, without a teacher to lead or cue your every move, you need your own little pot of knowledge from which you can scoop out ideas for your self-practice. Knowledge of both the yoga side of things, and of yourself and your body.

Note I said **little** here. You **do not** need to:

o Know an exhaustive list of yoga postures off the top of your head
o Know everything there is to know about how those postures work
o Know all there is to know about your body type and how to modify postures to suit it
o Have your own yoga teacher on tap
o Ever feel doubt or awkwardness when you step on your mat

This is going to vary for each of us. Partly, this is about confidence. Some will feel ready having taken a handful of online classes. For others it may take years of going to regular studio classes before they even consider rolling out a mat at home.

However, it is also about how developed your practice is. Especially when it comes to a Vinyasa self-practice. Let's talk a bit more about this . . .

How to know if you are ready for a Vinyasa self-practice:

In class, I can follow along most of the time when only hearing the cue for the postures.

I can do Sun Salutation A and Sun Salutation B without being cued.[1]

I am beginning to understand my own body type and anatomy. [2]

I am aware of how to adjust and modify my practice to reflect this but am always keen to learn more. [3]

I have resources I can check, or people to reach out to who can help me learn more about asana and my body as I continue to practice: be it an in-person class or teacher or friend, an online class or community, or books to read.

I know this process of learning and practicing is ongoing and that I am NEVER going to know everything there is to know about yoga or my body.

---

1. It's ok to have to check in with a reference source before you practice

2. For example: that I have tight hamstrings, or that my wrists need protecting, or that I tend to let my front knee lean in in warrior postures

3. If I have tight hamstrings, I bend my knees in a forward fold, for example

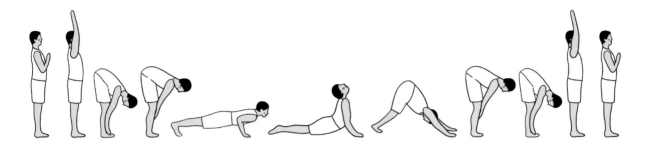

If you identify with most of these statements, I'd bet you are ready to give your self-practice a proper go!

Self-practice is a journey. You may be right at the start of it, and that's ok.

"

At once, there is nothing new
and yet no one has ever lived
what you are about to live.
This is a timeless paradox.

-

Mark Nepo

"

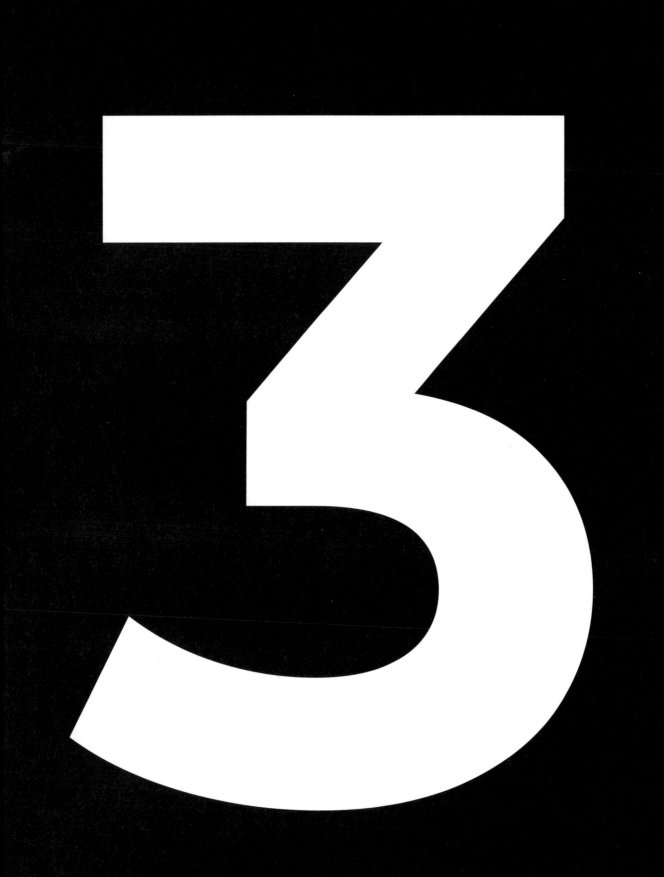

Getting on Your Mat

Asanas:
Dynamic internal dances in the form of postures. These help to keep the body strong, flexible, and relaxed.

Their practice strengthens the nervous system and refines our process of inner perception.

-

Donna Farhi

The
WHAT

How Do I Know What to Practice?

Anyone who has tried a self-practice has been there ... alone on your mat, with not one single clue of what to do.

It is a lonely and disheartening place. So much so that even the thought of it puts many of us off getting on that mat in the first place.

These first five tools are designed to help you build your own reference library of inspiration so that this fear is much more rare.

"

Move your joints every day. You have to find your own tricks. Bury your mind deep in your heart, and watch the body move by itself.

-

Sri Dharma Mittra

"

These five tools will help you find **what** you want to practice.

They can be used all together, individually, or mixed and matched.

They are the tools; **you** are the maker.

Tool #1

The Pose Selector

Tool #2

The Idea Generator

Tool #3

Beats

Tool #4

Breath

Tool #5

Tuning In

#1

—

The Pose Selector

This is how you approach the overwhelming number of postures there are in yoga. **The idea is to use it as a jump-off point for a practice.**

You will find a list of poses on pages 70–75. Take one heading or take a few specific poses (two or three are normally enough) with you onto your mat.

It is NOT an exhaustive list of all postures, and it is NOT a sequence builder. If this is what you are looking for then there are lots of amazing compendiums of yoga postures out there: books, apps, eBooks, all sorts.

However, in my humble opinion, these will not be that helpful to build your self-practice on. Most contain hundreds if not thousands of postures. And you know what happens to the human brain when confronted with thousands of options? It shuts down.

Instead, The Pose Selector is here to get you thinking about poses in various buckets in order to enable you to use the knowledge you have already in a practical fashion.

Maybe you know what part of your body you want to focus on in your practice but need some ideas for new poses in order to try something different.

Maybe you want to deepen your practice within a certain pose category but want to work on poses you wouldn't normally choose. Maybe you want to dedicate your practice to a type of postures you would never normally do. THAT is what The Pose Selector is here for.

It is also a template for you to use to jot down poses that spring up in your practice which you sometimes (or often!) forget.

Understanding the Three Sections:

The Pose Selector is broken down into three parts:

1. **Pose Type**
2. **Body Parts**
3. **Peak Poses**

Sore back from working at a desk all day? You are a keen cyclist or runner and want to address the imbalance by working on your arms?

Want to work on your backbends so you can start to flip your grip in certain postures? These are very natural ways we approach our practice with a purpose in mind.

By having prompts for a practice by BODY PART and by POSE TYPE we have a bunch of potential practices at our fingertips. These top-level prompts can also remind us of areas we might naturally neglect in our practices (when was the last time you did an entire practice focused on twists for example?!).

What is a Peak Pose?

A PEAK POSE is simply a pose you want to focus on specifically in your practice. Working towards a peak pose is a great way to progress your practice over the long term. It forces you to think about all the component parts you need to spend time on in order to reach that pose safely and when you are truly ready. This means it is an amazing way to build an in-depth understanding of more complex postures and how your own body works.

Peak poses DO NOT have to be advanced. Downward facing dog is an amazing peak pose: try holding it for 3 minutes and tell me that's not some of the hardest work you've done in a long while! You will have wanted to work on your shoulder strength and external rotation, as well as hamstring lengthening before that wouldn't you?

The 12 Peak Pose examples on page 70 are broken down into a Pose Type and two Body Part categories. You can then use the right parts of the Pose Selector to help you come up with poses to focus on before you get to your Peak Pose.

Building out your own Pose Selector

At the end of this book, in the Templates section on page 280, you will find blank versions of The Pose Selector which you can use to build this tool out to be totally bespoke to you.

Add new postures as you learn them, or old ones you may have forgotten. Create lists of all your favourites that you are shocked I am missing. Jot down fresh ideas for approaching Peak Poses that a teacher has shared with you. Use this tool and these templates as a personal library and you will never be short of practice ideas again.

Posture Naming Conventions in this Book

You will find both the English and Sanskrit names for postures in this section. While in the body of the text of this book, poses are just called by their English names for readability. I would STRONGLY encourage you as you progress through your yoga journey to learn the Sanskrit names for poses. The Sanskrit glossary on pages 270–273 is here to help with this. Yoga is an ancient Indian practice, and using Sanskrit is one way of honouring this.

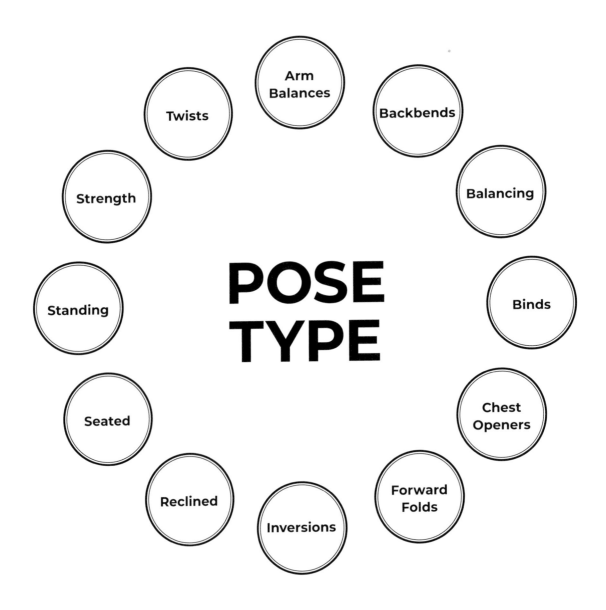

POSE TYPE

Arm Balances

Backbends

Balancing

Binds

Chest Openers

Forward Folds

Inversions

Reclined

Seated

Standing

Strength

Twists

Arm Balances

Chinstand: *Ganda Bherundasana*
Crane: *Kakasana*
Crow: *Bakasana*
Eight-Angle: *Astavakrasana*
EPK 1: *Eka Pada Koundinyanasana I*
EPK 2: *Eka Pada Koundinyanasana II*
Fallen Angel:
Devaduuta Panna Asana
Firefly: *Tittibhasana*
Flying Warrior: *Visvamitrasana*
Peacock: *Mayurasana*
Pendant: *Lolasana*
Scale: *Tolasana*
Shoulder-Pressing: *Bhujapidasana*
Side Crane (Crow): *Parsva Bakasana*
Yoga Push-Up:
Chaturanga Dandasana

Backbends

Bow: *Dhanurasana*
Bridge: *Setu Bandha Sarvangasana*
Camel: *Ustrasana*
Cobra: *Bhujangasana*
Cow: *Bitilasana*
Dancer's: *Natarajasana*
Fish: *Matsyasana*
Forearm Wheel:
Dwi Pada Viparita Dandasana
King Pigeon: *Kapotasana*
Locust: *Salabhasana*
One-Legged King Pigeon:
Eka Pada Rajakapotasana
One-Legged King Pigeon II:
Eka Pada Rajakapotasana II
Sphinx: *Salamba Bhujangasana*
Tiger: *Vyaghrasana*
Upward-Facing Dog:
Urdhva Mukha Svanasana
Wheel: *Urdhva Dhanurasana*
Wild Thing: *Camatkarasana*

Balancing

Bird of Paradise: *Svarga Dvidasana*
Dancer's: *Natarajasana*
Eagle: *Garudasana*
Extended Hand-to-Big-Toe:
Utthita Hasta Padangustasana
Half Moon: *Ardha Chandrasana*
Handstand: *Adho Mukha Vrksasana*
Headstand: *Sirsasana*
Side Plank: *Vasisthasana*
Tree: *Vrksasana*
Warrior III: *Virabhadrasana III*

Binds

Bird of Paradise: *Svarga Dvidasana*
Bound Extended Side Angle:
Baddha Parsvakonasana
Compass:
Parivrtta Surya Yantrasana
Half Bound Lotus Standing
Forward Bend:
Ardha Baddha Padmottanasana
Noose: *Pasasana*
Sage's 1: *Marichyasana I*
Sage's 3: *Marichyasana III*
Sugarcane: *Chapasana*
Super Soldier:
Viparita Parivrtta Surya Yantrasana
Tiger: *Vyaghrasana*

Chest Openers

Bow: *Dhanurasana*
Camel: *Ustrasana*
Cow: *Bitilasana*
Dancer's: *Natarajasana*
Extended Side Angle:
Utthita Parsvakonasana
Fish: *Matsyasana*
Forearm Wheel:
Dwi Pada Viparita Dandasana
Sphinx: *Salamba Bhujangasana*
Upward-Facing Dog:
Urdhva Mukha Svanasana
Wheel: *Urdhva Dhanurasana*
Wild Thing: *Camatkarasana*

Forward Folds

Child's: *Balasana*
Head-to-Knee Forward Bend:
Janu Sirsasana
Humble Warrior:
Baddha Virabhadrasana
Intense Side Stretch:
Parsvottanasana
Sage's 1: *Marichyasana I*
Seated Forward Bend:
Paschimottanasana
Standing Forward Bend: *Uttanasana*
Standing Half Forward Bend:
Ardha Uttanasana
Standing Split:
Urdhva Prasarita Eka Padasana
Tortoise: *Kurmasana*
Wide-Angle Seated Forward Bend:
Upavistha Konasana
Wide-Legged Forward Bend:
Prasarita Padottanasana

Inversions

Dolphin: *Ardha Pincha Mayurasana*
Downward-Facing Dog:
Adho Mukha Svanasana
Forearm Stand: *Pincha Mayurasana*
Handstand: *Adho Mukha Vrksasana*
Headstand: *Sirsasana*
Legs-Up-the-Wall: *Viparita Karani*
Plough: *Halasana*
Supported Shoulderstand:
Salamba Sarvangasana

Reclined

Fish: *Matsyasana*
Happy Baby: *Ananda Balasana*
Reclined Butterfly:
Supta Baddha Konasana
Reclined Pigeon / Eye of the Needle:
Supta Kapotasana
Reclined Twist:
Supta Matsyendrasana
Reclining Hand-to-Big-Toe:
Supta Padangusthasana
Reclining Hero: *Supta Virasana*

Seated

Boat: *Paripurna Navasana*
Bound Angle: *Baddha Konasana*
Compass:
Parivrtta Surya Yantrasana
Cow Face: *Gomukhasana*
Easy: *Sukhasana*
Fire Log / Double Pigeon:
Agnistambhasana
Half Lord of the Fishes:
Ardha Matsyendrasana
Head-to-Knee Forward Bend:
Janu Sirsasana
Hero: *Virasana*
Heron: *Krounchasana*
Lotus: *Padmasana*
Revolved Head-to-Knee:
Parivrtta Janu Sirsasana
Sage's 3: *Marichyasana III*
Seated Forward Bend:
Paschimottanasana
Splits: *Hanumanasana*
Staff: *Dandasana*
Wide-Angle Seated Forward Bend:
Upavistha Konasana

Standing

Big Toe: *Padangusthasana*
Bird of Paradise: *Svarga Dvidasana*
Chair: *Utkatasana*
Crescent: *Anjaneyasana*
Eagle: *Garudasana*
Extended Hand-to-Big-Toe:
Utthita Hasta Padangustasana
Extended Side Angle:
Utthita Parsvakonasana
Extended Triangle:
Utthita Trikonasana
Gate: *Parighasana*
Goddess: *Utkata Konasana*
Half Moon: *Ardha Chandrasana*
High Lunge:
Utthita Ashwa Sanchalanasana
Humble Warrior:
Baddha Virabhadrasana
Intense Side Stretch:
Parsvottanasana
Low Lunge: *Anjaneyasana*
Mountain: *Tadasana*
Revolved Side Angle:
Parivrtta Parsvakonasana
Revolved Triangle:
Parivrtta Trikonasana
Side Lunge: *Skandasana*

Standing Half Forward Bend:
Ardha Uttanasana
Standing Split:
Urdhva Prasarita Eka Padasana
Tree: *Vrksasana*
Upward Salute: *Urdhva Hastasana*
Warrior I: *Virabhadrasana I*
Warrior II: *Virabhadrasana II*

Strength

Boat: *Paripurna Navasana*
Chair: *Utkatasana*
Dolphin: *Ardha Pincha Mayurasana*
Downward-Facing Dog:
Adho Mukha Svanasana
Extended Side Angle:
Utthita Parsvakonasana
Extended Triangle:
Utthita Trikonasana
Forearm Plank:
Makara Adho Mukha Svanasana
Forearm Stand:
Pincha Mayurasana
Handstand: *Adho Mukha Vrksasana*
Locust: *Salabhasana*
Plank: *Kumbhakasana*
Reverse Plank: *Purvottanasana*
Revolved Side Angle:
Parivrtta Parsvakonasana
Revolved Triangle:
Parivrtta Trikonasana
Scale: *Tolasana*
Shoulder-Pressing: *Bhujapidasana*
Side Plank: *Vasisthasana*
Warrior I: *Virabhadrasana I*
Warrior II: *Virabhadrasana II*
Warrior III: *Virabhadrasana III*
Wheel: *Urdhva Dhanurasana*
Wide-Legged Forward Bend:
Prasarita Padottanasana
Yogi Push-Up:
Chaturanga Dandasana
Yogi Squat: *Malasana*

Twists

EPK 1: *Eka Pada Koundinyanasana I*
Half Lord of the Fishes:
Ardha Matsyendrasana
Noose: *Pasasana*
Revolved Head-to-Knee:
Parivrtta Janu Sirsasana
Revolved Side Angle:
Parivrtta Parsvakonasana
Revolved Triangle: *Parivrtta Trikonasana*
Sage's 3: *Marichyasana III*

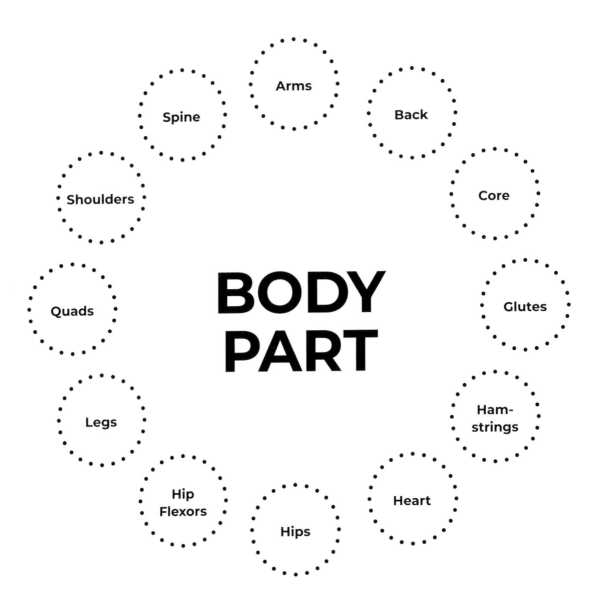

BODY PART

Arms

Back

Core

Glutes

Ham-
strings

Heart

Hips

Hip
Flexors

Legs

Quads

Shoulders

Spine

Arms

Crane (Crow): *Bakasana*
Dolphin: *Ardha Pincha Mayurasana*
Downward-Facing Dog:
Adho Mukha Svanasana
Eight-Angle: *Astavakrasana*
EPK 1: *Eka Pada Koundinyanasana I*
EPK 2: *Eka Pada Koundinyanasana II*
Firefly: *Tittibhasana*
Forearm Plank:
Makara Adho Mukha Svanasana
Forearm Stand: *Pincha Mayurasana*
Handstand: *Adho Mukha Vrksasana*
Headstand: *Sirsasana*
Peacock: *Mayurasana*
Plank: *Kumbhakasana*
Side Crane (Crow): *Parsva Bakasana*
Side Plank: *Vasisthasana*
Upward Salute: *Urdhva Hastasana*
Upward-Facing Dog:
Urdhva Mukha Svanasana
Wheel: *Urdhva Dhanurasana*
Wild Thing: *Camatkarasana*
Yogi Push-Up: *Chaturanga Dandasana*

Back

Bridge: *Setu Bandha Sarvangasana*
Cat: *Marjaryasana*
Cobra: *Bhujangasana*
Cow: *Bitilasana*
Head-to-Knee Forward Bend:
Janu Sirsasana
Locust: *Salabhasana*
Peacock: *Mayurasana*
Seated Forward Bend:
Paschimottanasana
Sphinx: *Salamba Bhujangasana*
Staff: *Dandasana*
Standing Half Forward Bend:
Ardha Uttanasana
Supported Shoulderstand:
Salamba Sarvangasana
Upward-Facing Dog:
Urdhva Mukha Svanasana
Yogi Squat: *Malasana*

Core

Boat: *Paripurna Navasana*
Chair: *Utkatasana*
Crow: *Bakasana*
Forearm Plank:
Makara Adho Mukha Svanasana
Pendant: *Lolasana*
Plank: *Kumbhakasana*
Scale: *Tolasana*
Side Plank: *Vasisthasana*
Yogi Push-Up: *Chaturanga Dandasana*

Glutes

Bridge: *Setu Bandha Sarvangasana*
Goddess: *Utkata Konasana*
Locust: *Salabhasana*
Mountain: *Tadasana*
Reverse Plank: *Purvottanasana*
Supported Shoulderstand:
Salamba Sarvangasana
Yogi Squat: *Malasana*

Hamstrings

Big Toe: *Padangusthasana*
Downward-Facing Dog:
Adho Mukha Svanasana
EPK 2:
Eka Pada Koundinyanasana II
Extended Hand-to-Big-Toe:
Utthita Hasta Padangustasana
Extended Triangle: *Utthita Trikonasana*
Firefly: *Tittibhasana*
Gate: *Parighasana*
Head-to-Knee Forward Bend:
Janu Sirsasana
Intense Side Stretch:
Parsvottanasana
Locust: *Salabhasana*
Reclining Hand-to-Big-Toe:
Supta Padangusthasana
Revolved Head-to-Knee: Parivrtta
Janu Sirsasana
Sage's 1: *Marichyasana I*
Seated Forward Bend:
Paschimottanasana
Splits: *Hanumanasana*
Staff: *Dandasana*
Standing Forward Bend:
Uttanasana
Standing Split:
Urdhva Prasarita Eka Padasana
Wide-Angle Seated Forward Bend:
Upavistha Konasana
Wide-Legged Forward Bend:
Prasarita Padottanasana

Heart

Bridge: *Setu Bandha Sarvangasana*
Cat: *Marjaryasana*
Cobra: *Bhujangasana*
Extended Puppy: *Uttana Shishosana*
King Pigeon: *Kapotasana*
Reclining Bound Angle:
Supta Baddha Konasana
Reverse Plank: *Purvottanasana*
Staff: *Dandasana*

Hips

Bound Angle: *Baddha Konasana*
Child's: *Balasana*
Cow Face: *Gomukhasana*
Eagle: *Garudasana*
Easy: *Sukhasana*
Extended Hand-to-Big-Toe:
Utthita Hasta Padangustasana
Extended Triangle: *Utthita Trikonasana*
Fire Log / Double Pigeon:
Agnistambhasana
Frog: *Bhekasana*
Goddess: *Utkata Konasana*
Half Moon: *Ardha Chandrasana*
Happy Baby: *Ananda Balasana*
Heron: *Krounchasana*
Humble Warrior:
Baddha Virabhadrasana
Lotus: *Padmasana*
One-Legged King Pigeon:
Eka Pada Rajakapotasana
One-Legged King Pigeon II:
Eka Pada Rajakapotasana II
Reclining Bound Angle:
Supta Baddha Konasana
Sage's 1: *Marichyasana I*

Sage's 3: *Marichyasana III*
Side Lunge: *Skandasana*
Tortoise: *Kurmasana*
Tree: *Vrksasana*
Wide-Angle Seated Forward Bend:
Upavistha Konasana
Wide-Legged Forward Bend:
Prasarita Padottanasana
Yogi Squat: *Malasana*

Hip Flexors

Boat: *Paripurna Navasana*
Bow: *Dhanurasana*
Bridge: *Setu Bandha Sarvangasana*
Camel: *Ustrasana*
Crow: *Bakasana*
Crescent: *Anjaneyasana*
Eight-Angle: *Astavakrasana*
Fish: *Matsyasana*
High Lunge:
Utthita Ashwa Sanchalanasana
King Pigeon: *Kapotasana*
Low Lunge: *Anjaneyasana*
One-Legged King Pigeon II:
Eka Pada Rajakapotasana II
Reclining Hero: *Supta Virasana*
Scale: *Tolasana*
Shoulder-Pressing: *Bhujapidasana*
Side Crow: *Parsva Bakasana*
Splits: *Hanumanasana*
Upward-Facing Dog:
Urdhva Mukha Svanasana

Legs

Big Toe: *Padangusthasana*
Downward-Facing Dog:
Adho Mukha Svanasana
Extended Side Angle:
Utthita Parsvakonasana
Extended Triangle:
Utthita Trikonasana
High Lunge:
Utthita Ashwa Sanchalanasana
Humble Warrior:
Baddha Virabhadrasana
Intense Side Stretch:
Parsvottanasana
Legs-Up-the-Wall: *Viparita Karani*
Mountain: *Tadasana*
Revolved Triangle:
Parivrtta Trikonasana
Staff: *Dandasana*
Standing Forward Bend:
Uttanasana
Tree: *Vrksasana*
Upward Salute: *Urdhva Hastasana*
Warrior 2 & 3: *Virabhadrasana II & III*
Wheel: *Urdhva Dhanurasana*

Quads

Camel: *Ustrasana*
Chair: *Utkatasana*
Child's: *Balasana* .
Crescent: *Anjaneyasana*
Dancer's: *Natarajasana*
Forearm Wheel:
Dwi Pada Viparita Dandasana
Half Frog: *Ardha Bhekasana*
Hero: *Virasana*
High Lunge:
Utthita Ashwa Sanchalanasana

King Pigeon: *Kapotasana*
Locust: *Salabhasana*
Low Lunge: *Anjaneyasana*
One-Legged King Pigeon:
Eka Pada Rajakapotasana
One-Legged King Pigeon II:
Eka Pada Rajakapotasana II
Reclining Bound Angle:
Supta Baddha Konasana
Reclining Hand-to-Big-Toe:
Supta Padangusthasana
Reclining Hero: *Supta Virasana*
Reverse Plank: *Purvottanasana*
Splits: *Hanumanasana*
Staff: *Dandasana*
Standing Split:
Urdhva Prasarita Eka Padasana
Sugarcane: *Chapasana*
Warrior I: *Virabhadrasana I*
Warrior II: *Virabhadrasana II*

Shoulders

Bow: *Dhanurasana*
Cat: *Marjaryasana*
Dancer's: *Natarajasana*
Dolphin: *Ardha Pincha Mayurasana*
Eagle: *Garudasana*
Extended Puppy: *Uttana Shishosana*
Firefly: *Tittibhasana*
Forearm Plank:
Makara Adho Mukha Svanasana
Forearm Stand: *Pincha Mayurasana*
Forearm Wheel:
Dwi Pada Viparita Dandasana
Handstand: *Adho Mukha Vrksasana*
Noose: *Pasasana*
Plow: *Halasana*
Reverse Plank: *Purvottanasana*
Revolved Head-to-Knee:
Parivrtta Janu Sirsasana
Revolved Side Angle:
Parivrtta Parsvakonasana
Revolved Triangle:
Parivrtta Trikonasana
Sage's 1: *Marichyasana I*
Sage's 3: *Marichyasana III*
Side Plank: *Vasisthasana*
Supported Shoulderstand:
Salamba Sarvangasana

Spine

Bow: *Dhanurasana*
Camel: *Ustrasana*
Cat: *Marjaryasana*
Cobra: *Bhujangasana*
Fish: *Matsyasana*
Forearm Wheel:
Dwi Pada Viparita Dandasana
Gate: *Parighasana*
Half Lord of the Fishes:
Ardha Matsyendrasana
Intense Side Stretch:
Parsvottanasana
Lotus: *Padmasana*
Revolved Head-to-Knee:
Parivrtta Janu Sirsasana
Seated Forward Bend:
Paschimottanasana
Wheel: *Urdhva Dhanurasana*
Wide-Legged Forward Bend:
Prasarita Padottanasana
Wild Thing: *Camatkarasana*

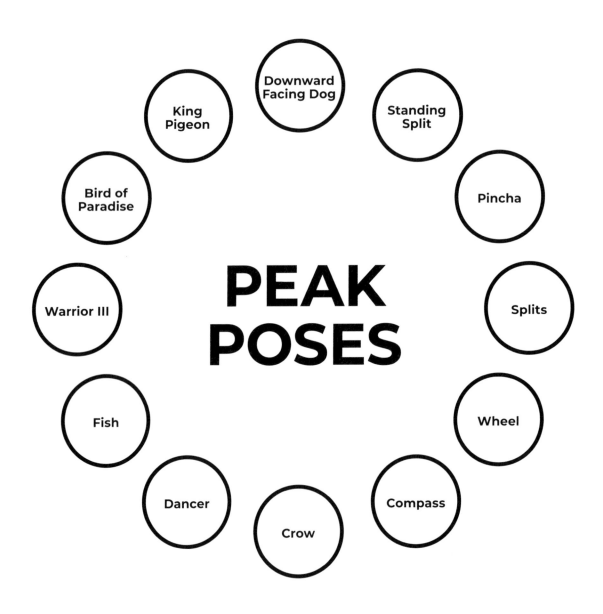

PEAK POSES

Downward Facing Dog

Standing Split

Pincha

Splits

Wheel

Compass

Crow

Dancer

Fish

Warrior III

Bird of Paradise

King Pigeon

Peak Pose	Pose Type	Body Part	
Downward-Facing Dog *Adho Mukha Svanasana*	Strength	Shoulders	Hamstrings
Standing Split *Urdhva Prasarita Eka Padasana*	Forward Fold	Hamstrings	Hips
Forearm Stand *Pincha Mayurasana*	Inversion	Arms	Shoulders
Splits *Hanumanasana*	Seated	Legs	Hip Flexors
Wheel *Urdhva Dhanurasana*	Backbend	Glutes	Heart
Compass *Parivrtta Surya Yantrasana*	Twist	Heart	Core
Crow *Bakasana*	Arm Balance	Core	Arms
Dancer's *Natarajasana*	Standing	Spine	Legs
Fish *Matsyasana*	Reclined	Quads	Back
Warrior III *Virabhadrasana III*	Balancing	Back	Legs
Bird of Paradise *Svarga Dvidasana*	Bind	Hips	Hamstrings
King Pigeon *Kapotasana*	Chest Opener	Hip Flexors	Heart

#2

The Idea Generator

Pick one idea from this tool, apply it as you practice, and see how your default yoga is transformed

The concept here is that each one-liner is incredibly easy to hold in your head as you practice.

And that one line will prompt your mind and body to find something new in the postures and in the sequences they already know.

One of the blissful elements of taking a led class is the surprise of not knowing what is coming next, and, if you have a good teacher, imaginative and inspired sequencing. No one wants to trog through the same boring Warrior II – Reverse Warrior – Extended Side Angle sequence again and again do they?!

The Idea Generator works especially well if you are taking something from The Pose Selector as the foundation for your practice. How would your backbend practice feel if you put your elbows down on your mat instead of your hands? What would a hamstring focused practice feel like if you held every posture for five breaths? What would a Sun Salutation B look like if you added a bind to every posture?

It's not rocket science. But neither is yoga! Add a wiggle to Warrior II. Lift up to your tip toes in Chair pose. Hook that free hand onto your body where you can. Anything is possible. And this is the tool to help you discover those possibilities.

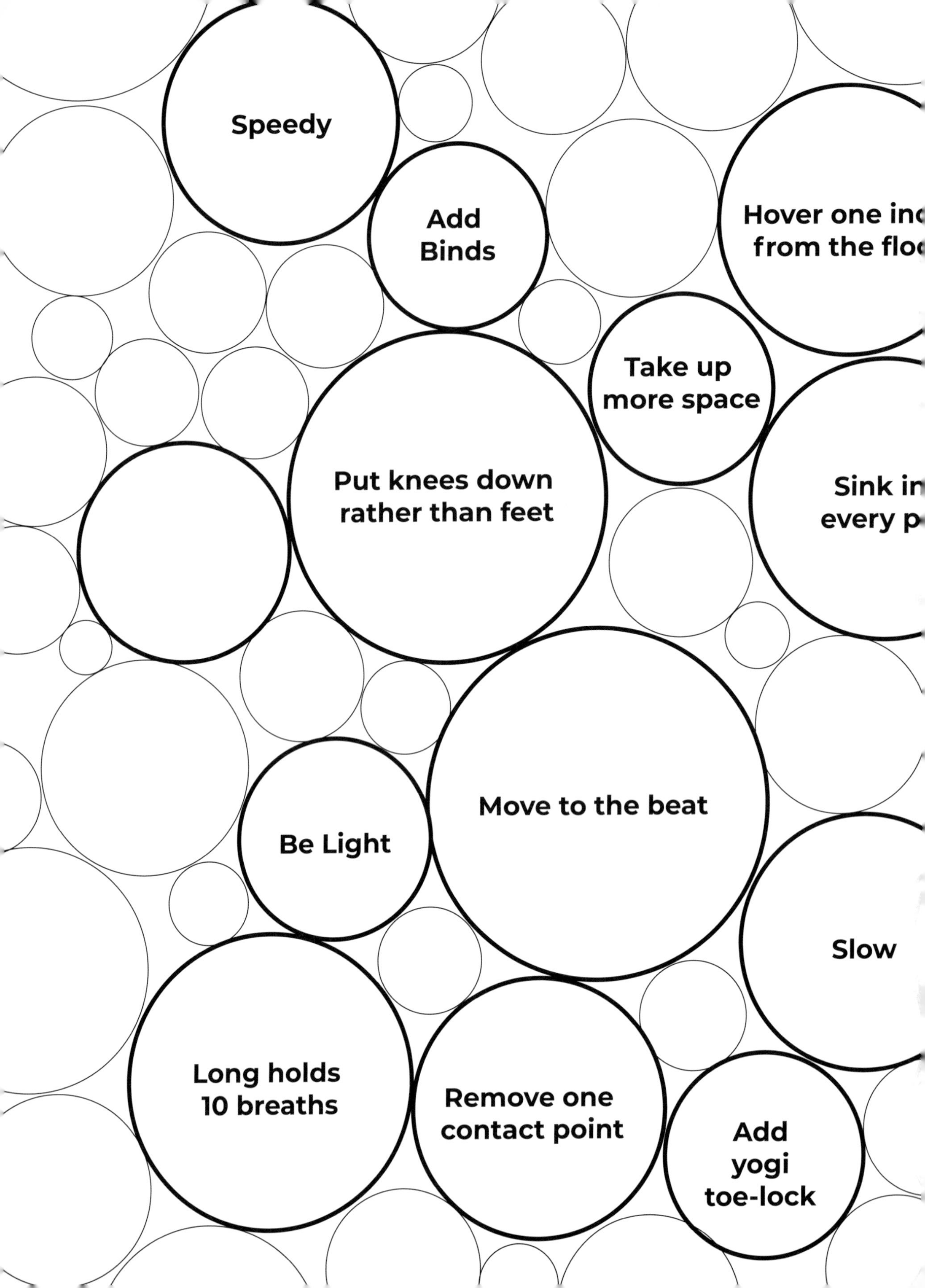
Speedy
Add Binds
Hover one in
from the flo
Take up more space
Put knees down rather than feet
Sink in
every p
Move to the beat
Be Light
Slow
Long holds 10 breaths
Remove one contact point
Add yogi toe-lock

Put elbows down rather than hands

One Fast
One Slow

Long holds
5 breaths

Widen
Everything

Close
your eyes

Articulate
your spine

3 of each

Move only to
your breath

On tip toes

Add one
contact point

One breath
one movement

Take up
less space

The Idea Generator

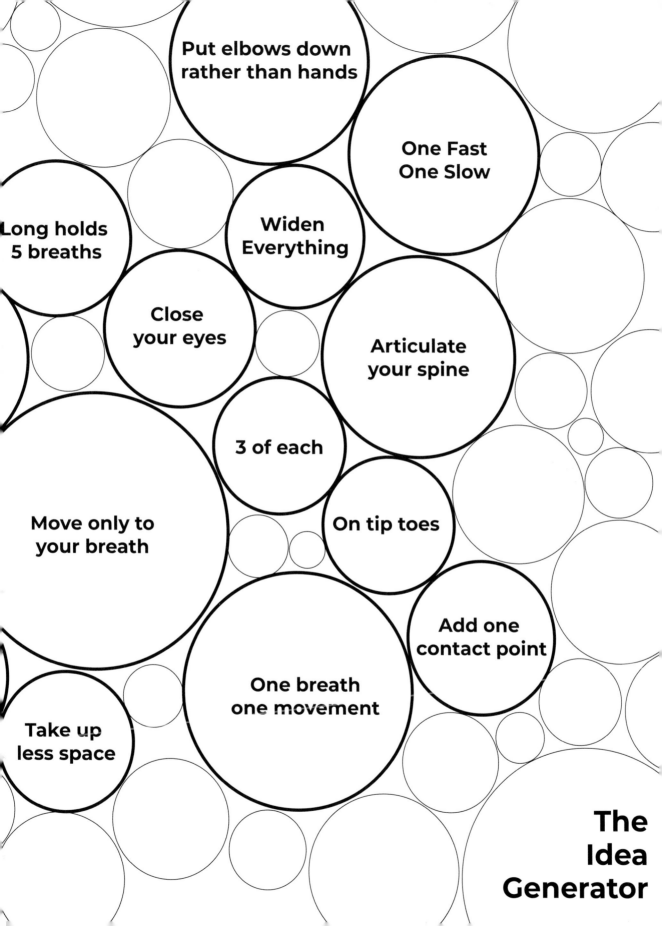

#3
—

Beats

Music can be such a powerful influence on our emotions and movements. Use that to your advantage when you practice. Curating playlists tends to be a love or hate exercise for people: so, pick your poison . . .

If you hate it . . . use the experts.
Don't feel like you have to reinvent the wheel. Many, MANY people who love music more, or who have more time or incentive to craft great music selections have already done so. All you have to do is find them!

And this is where services like Spotify and SoundCloud come into their own.

Do you go to a class where the teacher always plays the perfect music? Ask them if you can listen to it anywhere.

Do you follow yogis on Instagram or YouTube who pick amazing tunes? Ask them if they share their playlists anywhere.

If you love it . . . build your own
This can be a quick and easy task, or a much more involved one. It's totally up to you. If you love building playlists, here are some options that might work well for you.

1. The Power of Shuffle

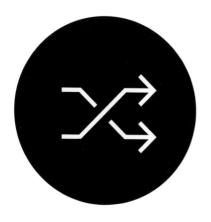

Whack all your favourite tunes onto one big playlist and press shuffle.

Sure, you might get a really upbeat track when you are warming up, and something more zen in the middle of your super dynamic Sun Salutation, but does it matter? No! You can skip a track. Or just keep going and either let the music guide you or carry on regardless.

2. Find the Beat

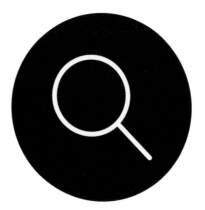

Have a couple of playlists (or more) which match the different types of practices you tend to go for.

Pumping tunes for the days when you want to get sweaty. And something calmer for the chilled out days.

3. The Wave Practice

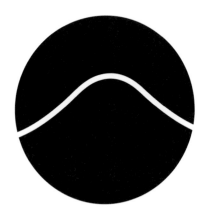

No idea what a Wave Practice is? Tool #9 on page 136 explains all.

For now, just know that this is your cheat-sheet for how to build a playlist which rises and falls with the intensity of a traditional Vinyasa-style practice.

The timings and numbers of songs are of course going to vary depending on how you like to flow and what kind of music you like to listen to. This is a starting point to work from, which you can adapt.

			Centre In & Warm Up	Sun Salutations	Main Sequences	Floor Sequence	Savasana
1	30 Min.	Time	5 min.	15 min.		7 min.	3 min.
		Songs	1–2	3–4		2	1
2	45 Min.	Time	5 min.	10 min.	15 min.	10 min.	5 min.
		Songs	1–2	2–3	3–4	2–3	1
3	60 Min.	Time	5 min.	15 min.	20 min.	15 min.	5 min.
		Songs	1–2	3–4	4–5	3–4	1
4	90 Min.	Time	10 min.	15 min.	35 min.	20 min.	10 min.
		Songs	2–3	3–4	6–8	4–5	2

Tips:

1. Choose soothing but uplifting songs that will tempt you to get going. If you are ever struggling to get on your mat you can press play on a playlist while still on the sofa. Then these warm-up songs will motivate you to begin.

2. Put your most upbeat tunes here. It can help to have a short, more chilled song in the transition between your Sun Salutations and the main sequence so you know where you are. Alternatively, place one halfway through your main sequence section to provide a rest or a signal to switch sides.

3. This is where to put those songs that inspire focus – meaningful lyrics or soaring melodies. You are likely to be holding postures for longer here, so pick songs that will help.

4. Try a small number of longer songs to minimise disruption to your Savasana.

4. Mix It Up

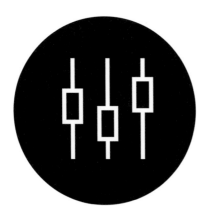

5. Sound of Silence

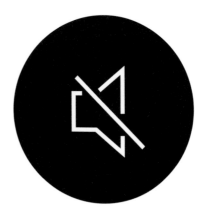

This is a great option for when you are stuck in a bit of a yoga rut and need to trick yourself into opening up and trying something new. Put on a genre of music you would never normally listen to, never mind practice to! Music with lyrics, music without lyrics, classical music, hip-hop, pop, Indian mantra ... Just see what happens. It might be a disaster, or it might be something special.

There is of course no need to listen to music at all when you practice. If you prefer silence, or the space it gives you to focus on your own breath, then great.

Again, this can be a really good approach for getting yourself out of your default practice.

#4
—
Breath

Use your breath to inspire and to transform your yoga practice.

Purists will probably be rolling their eyes that it's taken me 80 pages to get to the breath. Some have even defined yoga as being the marrying of movement and breath.

However, it can be a hurdle to new self-practitioners getting on their mat. It is an additional thing to worry you are getting 'wrong', especially when you are used to a teacher cueing you.

There is no right or wrong answer when it comes to breath and physical asana. Only what works for you.

Which might be very different things on different days, or at different points through your life.

There are yoga teachers that will disagree: their view is that 'correct' yogic breathing supports the movement or impact of the pose, and that 'incorrect' breathing has adverse effects. And to a certain extent they are right: you WILL find that working with your breath flows through to the ease with which you enter or hold postures, or how you move between them.

But you know what has more 'adverse effects' than breathing 'incorrectly', by which they mean the way that your body is naturally telling you at that moment? **Not doing yoga at all**.

If the hurdle is that you should only practice once you can do the breathing 'correctly' according to whoever the yoga police are, then guess what, very few of us are going to be practicing at all.

I would challenge anyone brand new to yoga to hold a Downward Facing Dog for a minute without breathing heavily (i.e. 'incorrectly'), no matter how hard they try to keep their breath effortless (i.e. 'correctly').

For someone who has been practicing for many years, they may need to be in a one-minute handstand to feel that same kind of focus and impact on their breath.

So … If thinking about your breathing helps you when you practice, then use it. If not, don't.

At the start, it's that simple. With time, and with practice, you will naturally start to focus more on your breath.

You will experience that you can reach both more deeply and more safely into a full forward fold with long smooth exhales. You will realise that you cannot hold that inversion with your breath held in tightly.

And hopefully with this tool you will start experimenting with how different types of breath can impact your practice.

Remember, the goal of each tool is to be a prompt to help your self-practice. Maybe this is one you use when you are getting bored of doing the same things most days and want to switch it up in a way you haven't done before. It may be that there is a type of breathing that you always want to use in your practice. Alternatively, try these different breaths when you want to engineer a different type of practice to your usual. Let's dive in a bit deeper to what the different types of conscious breath look like.

Deliberate vs. Natural Breath

When practicing yoga your breath can be either natural or deliberate.

With a Natural Breath, you simply breathe as you need to.

No pressure, no expectations, just prioritising whatever else it is you need to focus on in your practice today.

When you are in a relatively difficult posture or perhaps moving with more speed, you will be breathing more: more frequently, more deeply.

This is simply giving your body the oxygen it needs.

If this is your choice, then your goal can be to simply observe when those changes in your natural breath happen. Watch. And learn. It is still a breath you are aware of.

Alternatively, you can choose Deliberate Breath: consciously controlling the type of breath you are taking. Let's look at what that means in more detail …

In Vinyasa yoga, at a very general level, a different part of the breath is associated with different types of movement:

INHALE: expansive breaths match with expansive movements.

- When you open your body – particularly when opening the chest or heart.

- For any movement where the arms sweep up.

EXHALE: closing-in breaths match with closing-in movements.

- For forward folds – emptying the lungs means there is more room to find that compression between thighs and chest.

- For twists – emptying the lungs creates space and facilitates the movement.

Below is the classic Sun Salutation A along with inhale and exhale breath cues:

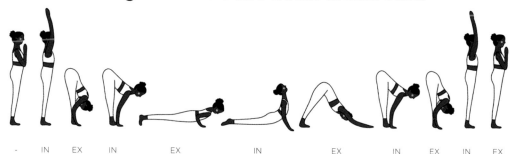

-     IN   EX   IN   EX   IN   EX   IN   EX   IN   EX

Deliberate Breath Types

When you are ready to get into a practice with a more deliberate breath, consider this spectrum of options:

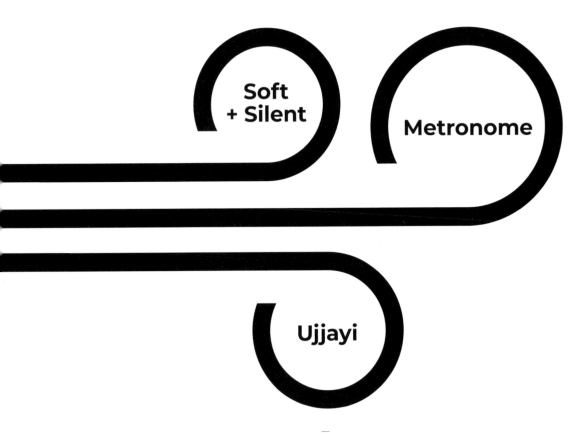

Soft and Silent Breathing

o A conscious breath but one where we try to make as little noise as possible. Even when the work is intense, there is effort to modulate the breath to keep it light, soft, and soundless.

o This comes most easily in slower, more gentle practices but can be an amazing additional challenge when paired with a super dynamic practice.

Metronome Breathing

o Where you count your breaths in your postures and transitions, or just your postures.

o Options include a simple one breath count for every posture/ transition in a sun salutation. Alternatively, hold every posture/ transition for a certain breath count: 3, 5, 10 or more.

o This can be a powerful choice for helping to quiet the mind and work on trickier postures or ones where you find yourself trying to 'get out' of them as soon as you have reached them. It's also a great option when you don't have music to practice to.

Ujjayi Breathing

o This is a breathing technique employed in a variety of yoga practices. It is sometimes called the 'ocean' breath or the 'victorious' breath. Many teachers will describe it as the breath you would make to fog up a mirror, but with your mouth closed. It tends to be done quite strongly: you'll know when someone next to you in a class is using it!

o It is most commonly associated with the Ashtanga method of yoga where there are precise breath instructions for every posture. As we naturally breathe more strongly when we are expending more effort, this breath also pairs naturally with other stronger types of practices such as dynamic Vinyasa.

o Adding a strong breath like this to a slower, calmer practice can bring a whole different experience to it.

#5

—

Tuning In

The skill of learning to listen to your body and letting that guide your practice.

Out of all the tools on the list, this is the one that can be used most powerfully on its own (though it can of course be used with the others as well).

It is also the hardest to teach. Especially to people like us: rushing around, striving, achieving, pushing on and on and on. So many, if not most, of us have never had to stop and listen to what messages our bodies are sending us. Our bodies are merely tools to facilitate the ambitions our brain has.

The very essence of yoga is this skill. It is why the physical practice of asana is such a core part of the philosophy:

being IN our bodies during our practice teaches us so much.

I'm going to keep it really simple here, with some questions that you can use to help you listen to what your body is already telling you.

Forgive me if this all seems obvious – it is – but I HAVE to be explicit about this tool as it is one we all so easily forget or ignore. That is until we injure ourselves, or get ill, and then everything comes grinding to a halt and we HAVE to listen.

Please don't wait for an external shock to force you to practice this skill and learn the deep lessons it will teach you.

Practice it now. Every day.

Notice I'm not saying 'every time you get on your mat'. Sometimes the answer that comes back from listening to your body will be not to do a physical practice at all. And that is ok. Actually it's more than ok. THAT is yoga.

Here are the four prompts to help you develop the skill of TUNING IN:

1. What is open/tight?
2. Am I feeling energetic/tired?
3. Do I want to lean in or ease off?
4. How do I do that in a way that feels right for me today?

Use these prompts to help you decide what postures or what type of practice to have today.

The
HOW

How do I Flow by Myself & Structure a Practice?

This next section is all about how to put the previous tools together: to form a flow, and to form a practice.

"

Since prana is energy and life force, pranayama means the extension and expansion of all our vital energy. It has to be clear you cannot just increase the volume of anything as volatile and explosive as pure energy without taking steps to contain, harness, and direct it ...

That is why Pantanjali clearly stated that between the practice of asana and pranayama, there is a step up. There has to exist, thought proficiency in asana, strength and stability in the circuitry of the body to withstand the increase in current that pranayama practice will bring.

-

B.K.S. Iyengar

"

What's the difference?

Flow:
Linking of one posture or asana to another.

This can be at any pace, holding the poses for any length of time, for as many or as few postures as you like.

The most well known of all Vinyasa flows is a Sun Salutation. Many yoga teachers and practitioners use the term 'vinyasa' itself to describe the connecting flow of moving from a posture like Downward Facing Dog to Chaturanga to Upward Facing Dog and back to Downward Dog.

The moment you move from one posture to another independently without a teacher telling you what to do, you have already created your own flow. It doesn't have to be fancy or complicated. **But if we want to keep returning to our mats then we do need our yoga practices to be INTERESTING.**

Practice:
A series of flows knitted together.

On some days this might just be a few short minutes; on others it might be hours. But any practice will have a basic structure: a beginning, a middle, and end. This can be as complicated or as simple as you like.

The first five tools in this book provided ideas for making the CONTENT of your flows, and therefore your practice, interesting and different.

The tools in this section will show you how to CREATIVELY knit those content ideas together in a way that makes sense for you, your body, and the time you have available. Because that is where things get really exciting.

Once you find your own inner creativity on your yoga mat, the limitless power of self-practice really gets unlocked.

These five tools will help you work out **how** to practice.

More than the other sections of the book, these tools should be read through sequentially.

Learn to flow without a teacher leading you, and then learn how to build these flows into a practice.

Creating a Flow

Tool #6

Hacking Sun Salutations

Tool #7

Change It Up

Tool #8

Creative Flows

Creating a Practice

Tool #9

The Wave Practice

Tool #10

The Mini Practice

Creating a Flow

A flow can be any number of postures linked together in any number of ways. But when the possibilities are limitless, we can start to feel overwhelmed.

These next tools will help you start simple, and then get more creative. Each has easy tricks that enable you to hold just one short sentence or cue in your mind as you move and let the flow develop spontaneously as you go from there. Sounds crazy?

Trust me, it works

Starting with Sun Salutations

The humble Sun Salutation or Surya Namaskār; the foundation of modern-day Vinyasa yoga.

There are 11 postures in the A variation, and 19 in the B; each pose flows from one to the next, in a continuous loop.

These two flows contain EVERYTHING you need to have a complete yoga asana practice: forward folds, backbends, inversions, core work, hip opening ... seriously everything.

Which is why we are going to use them as the basis for your independent vinyasa yoga practice. **Perhaps your first step is just learning these.**

Sun Salutation A

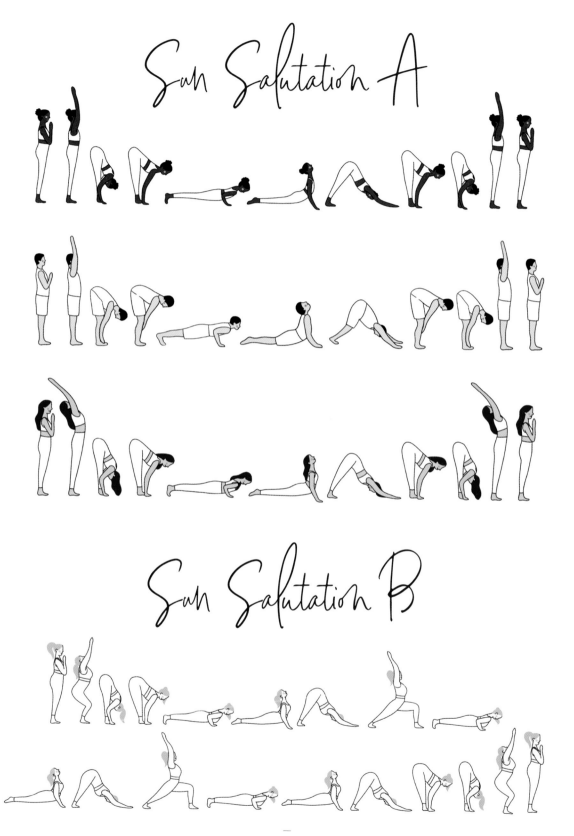

Sun Salutation B

6

Hacking Sun Salutations

How do you transform these set sequences into something of your very own? **You hack them.**

Once you know these sequences, then the next step is to use them as the basis for learning to flow creatively. All by yourself.

The power of using a sequence you already know to get creative is that you always have somewhere to go next or a point to come back to. Got lost? Go back to Downward Dog. Forgot what happens next?

Pick up at a point that is easy to get to. Totally lost your confidence? Simply start again.

Hacking Sun Salutations is all about working with what is already there, and then adding something of your own.

Another posture, a movement within a posture, a movement between postures:

anything goes.

Hacking Sun Sal A
Starting Out:

The easiest place to start with hacking a Sun Sal A is from your Downward Facing Dog.

Traditionally, this is where we take the most time in any of the postures in this flow, providing some time and space to THINK: what you can add in next, before returning to your Downward Dog and then completing the rest of the Sun Sal.

What should you add in? Anything you want – remember, this is what Tools #1 through to #5 are here to help with. Some postures or movements that would come to most of us trying this for the first time might be things like:

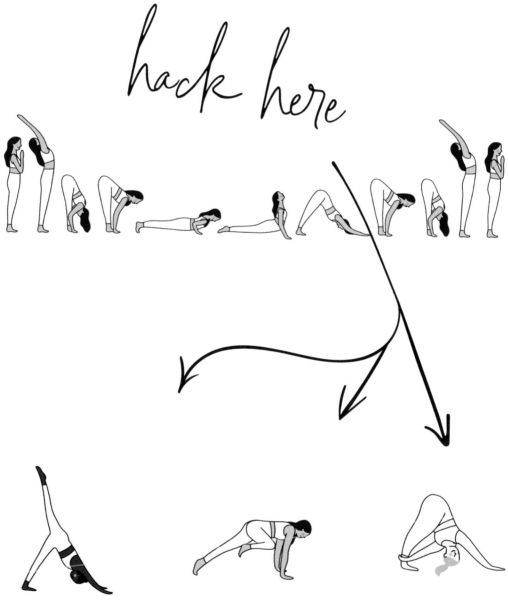

hack here

Three-Legged
Dog

Knee-to-Triceps
Reps

Revolved
Downward Dog

Hacking Sun Sal A
Getting Juicy:

Once you are super comfortable with hacking at that Downward Dog point, you can of course hack at any point in the flow.

Whatever you are adding in or trying, simply continue with the rest of your Sun Salutation afterwards and either add in the same thing as you move through the sequence again or try something else next time.

For example, you could:

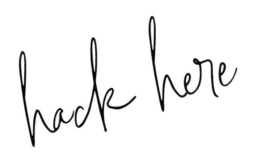

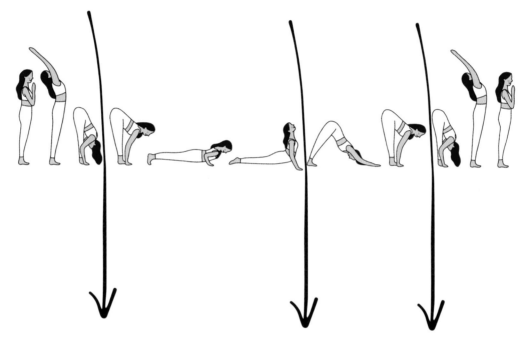

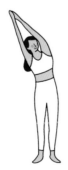

Add some side bends
in Mountain pose

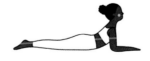

Move between Updog
and Sphinx pose 3 times

Work on your
Crow pose

Hacking Sun Sal B Starting Out:

The easiest place to hack your Sun Sal B is right before you hit Warrior I.

NOT from your Warrior I.

This is a small, but important distinction.

If you went to the world's most boring and unoriginal Vinyasa class, what would come next after Warrior I? Warrior II right? Then next? Reverse Warrior, no? And then next would be Extended Side Angle of course. And right after that you would be silently cursing your decision to pay money to attend this snoozefest of a class!

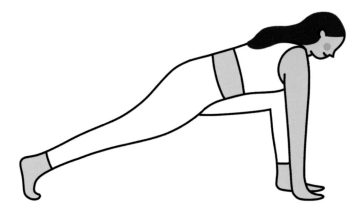

But let's be kind to this yoga teacher: once you are in your Warrior I it can feel like you are pretty committed to facing the front of your mat and continuing with standing postures.

However, if you put your 'hacking point' right before you get there, a world of other possibilities open up. In this high lunge shape, with your hands on the mat, it will feel like you have many more options. And you do! Why?

o Your weight is distributed across both hands and feet, so transferring it to any of these points feels natural and manageable.

o You are at the mid-height point on your mat, meaning kneeling, supine and standing postures are all easy to get to (the entire next tool is about how you can think about using these different heights, or planes, to jazz up your flows).

o Using this point as your jump-off point WILL mean you are more creative.

**Your Sun Sal
B will also get
hacked at two
points – on the
right-hand side,
and again on the
left-hand side.**

Add in anything
you want. Now
you have the
mechanics of
hacking your
Sun Salutations.

What comes next are the rules you
need to make sure this little trick
works for you.

Remember you are going to add your
new pose from the lunge you reach
before you get to your Warrior I. Here
are some postures or movements
that you can try:

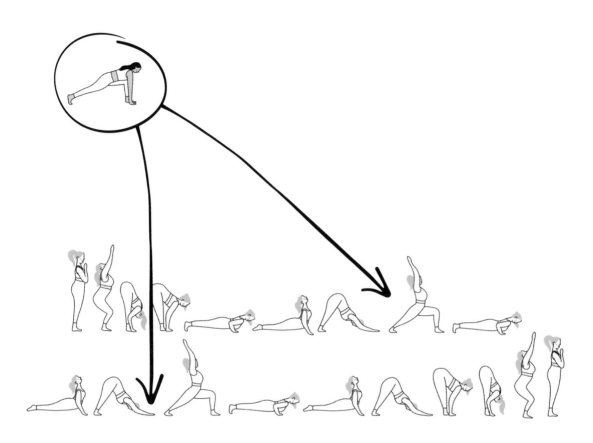

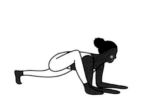

Lizard

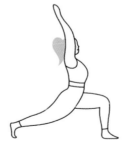

Lift up into a high lunge

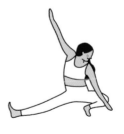

Rotate on the feet
to side lunge

Hacking Sun Sal B
Getting Juicy:

Once you are comfortable with hacking at that pre-Warrior I point, you are of course free to do so elsewhere in the flow. For example:

And your hacks here, or at any other point, don't need to be limited to one quick posture. You can add a few postures in, or a very long hold in one, or a little drill you have been working on. Give anything a try and see what brings you joy.

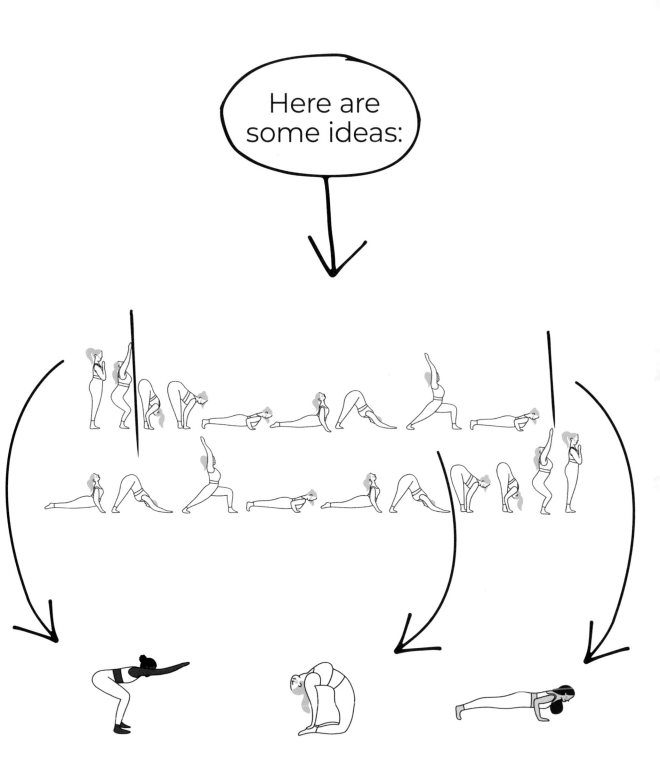

Here are some ideas:

10 second lower and hold in Half Chair

Lower knees and arch back to Camel

Chaturanga to Plank reps

Three Golden Rules of Yoga Hacking

1. Don't overload yourself:

Honestly, you are going to get embarrassed at how bad your memory can get when you are in the middle of a flow. You can be having a little panic about what comes next or having so much fun and being so present in your body on the first side that by the time the second side comes around you don't have the faintest clue what to do or what order to do it in!

This is ok! In fact, it's kind of the point. You want to have to practice getting comfortable with discomfort.

That tricky pose you add in will give you the practice with the physical discomfort. The challenge of adding and forgetting poses will give you practice of the mental discomfort.

These are the skills that you will take off your mat and that will have a profound impact on your life. Embrace the chance to practice them.

Start small so you don't scare yourself off: two, three or maximum four postures or movements is more than enough to keep things interesting.

2. Use Downward Facing Dog as thinking time:

This will be the most efficient thinking time of your entire day. Thinking time that gets into virtually every muscle in your body? Yes please!

Even if you are here for what feels like forever while you have a little ponder about what to do next, THAT'S OK.

Of course, any other pose you choose can work as well – Child's Pose is a personal favourite of mine.

3. Accept that perfection is your enemy:

The yoga police will not be storming into your bedroom to give you a telling off if you go astray mid-flow. You aren't going to permanently misalign your body by forgetting to do the same postures on the second side. You can stop halfway through a flow, take a few deep breaths and start all over again.

There is no perfection here. Only practice. Lots and lots and LOTS of practice.

#7

—

Change It Up

Interesting, varied and exciting practices can help bring us back to our mats again and again.

'Change It Up' will help you create flows that fit this bill totally on the fly. Yep, zero planning or prep. Just intuitively as you move.

You already have the tools to help with ideas for WHAT poses to do. And HOW & WHERE to hack your sun salutations. Now we are going to make your Sun Salutation 'hacks' more creative.

Simply by prompting yourself to change one thing:

1. Change Planes
2. Change Limbs
3. Change Direction

When you are asking yourself where to go next in your flow or how to put things together in an inventive way, just ask yourself: how can I change **Planes**, and/or change **Limbs**, and/or change **Direction**?

It's incredibly simple, you'll never forget it, and it always works. Let's go through some examples.

Change Planes

There are three planes in our yoga practice:

Low: lying on the mat

Medium: hands/knees on the mat

High: standing

The vast majority of yoga poses can be practiced on at least two planes, if not all three, in some variation.

By using this cue, you can take just one idea or one pose, and translate it into a stream of fresh postures, fresh flows, and therefore fresh feelings in your body and in your mind.

This change is the easiest one to start with: head back to your beginner Sun Salutation hacks (from Downward Facing Dog and from the low lunge right before your Warrior I) and see how this cue can inspire you to move into a posture you might never have chosen before.

These are some of my favourites:

Low
Lying on the mat

Medium
Hands/knees on the mat

High
Standing

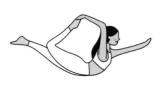

Half Bow

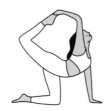

Tiger

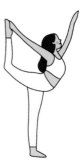

Dancers

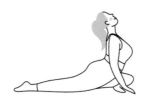

Pigeon

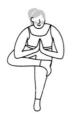

Figure Four

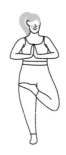

Standing Half Lotus

Change Limbs

It is natural once we have a leading leg or arm on a leading side to think that the next move has to be another pose that continues with that leading limb.

By cueing yourself to **change it**, you will automatically add more interest to your flow. Let's look at how this cue can inspire something different in your flows.

Here's a left leg leading example:

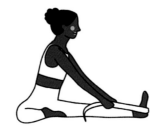

Seated Head-to-Knee pose

Change to right leg

Change to arm

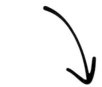

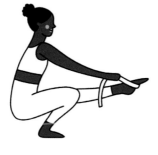

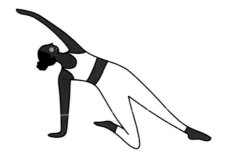

Place the right foot on the floor and lift up
to a Pistol Squat

Reach back with right hand to lift into Baby
Wild Thing

Change Direction

Exciting new things can happen in your practice if you flip one posture, or one part of your sequence towards a different direction on your mat.

Modern yoga mats are amazing inventions. With just the right amount of stickiness, a good mat makes the world of difference to a practice.

But while we all want a sticky mat, if you get stuck always facing 'the front' of your mat, you are going to have a harder time getting creativity and diversity into your practice.

Cue yourself to **change direction**:

Front to Back
Side to Side
Upright to Upside Down
Diagonal to Diagonal

Let's take something super simple, like a Warrior I and see how this cue can take you to new places.

So you are in your Warrior I:

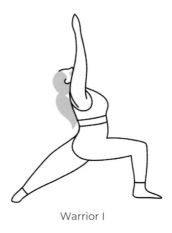

Warrior I

Upright to Upside Down

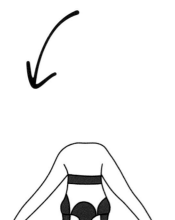

Rotate to the side for Wide-Legged
Forward Fold

Front to Back

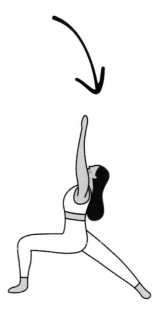

Spin around to face the 'back' of your mat,
hold the Warrior I and then continue your
Sun Salutation

#8
—

Creative
Flows

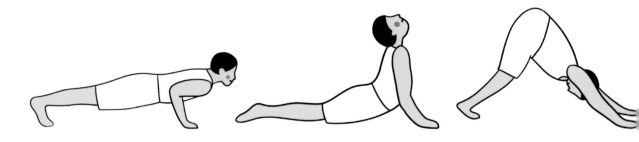

Ready to move beyond the set framework of Sun Salutations?

This tool empowers you to find complete creativity in your flows, in a neat and easy way, by setting a new RETURN POINT or finding a new CONNECTIING MINI-SEQUENCE.

Vinyasa is of course a style of yoga, but it is also the term many yoga teachers will use for the connecting sequence of Chaturanga to Upward Facing Dog to Downward Facing Dog.

This powerful little sequence can be used to link up different parts of your practice. But what if you are bored of vinyasas, done with endless Chaturangas, and never really liked Up Dog anyway? No worries! Pick a different return point, or a different connecting mini-sequence.

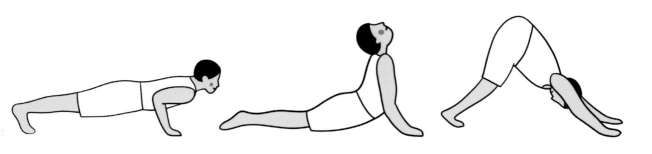

Return Point

A return point is a pose that you come back to – return to – once you have done your hacked Sun Salutation or come up with your own creative flow of postures.

It can separate your left-hand and right-hand side flows and be something you just visit briefly or hold for a longer period to time to develop your strength, flexibility, or knowledge that you can survive when the going gets tough!

Having a fresh return point really helps bring focus to your practice: it will give you lots of opportunities to come back to whatever it is you are working on. And by revisiting the pose again and again, you will start to observe and experience many more nuances than if it was just another pose in your flow.

Here are some suggestions:

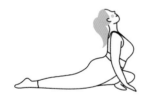

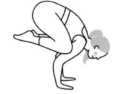

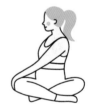

Hip Opening Flow:
you are flowing between lots of different hip opening postures, so add a long hold in Pigeon or Frog as your return point.

Strength Building Flow:
you are really working up a sweat and want to keep challenging yourself. Your return point could be a 10 breath hold in Crow.

Twist Focused Flow:
all your postures have a twisting adaptation, so return to a simple seated twist, turning both left and right to continue that theme.

Connecting
Mini Sequence:

Just as a traditional vinyasa can neatly book-end a creative sequence of postures, so too can any other mini-sequence.

A connecting mini-sequence is a small handful of postures that you will use throughout your practice to link one set of postures to another.

Centring it around the theme or focus of your practice, or a pose or skill or feeling you would like to engage deeper with works incredibly well too.

Let's build on the prior examples:

Hip Opening Flow

If a long hold in Pigeon or Frog doesn't fit with your dynamic practice today, then another option could be to flow like this:

 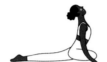

Strength Building Flow

Want to make that Crow Pose hold feel more flowy?
Then how about something like this?

   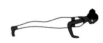

Twist Focused Flow

Building on our simple Seated Twist could look like this:

Creating a Practice

Now we get to put all of this together and create an entire standalone practice.

This is the moment when things can both be totally daunting and amazingly freeing! So embrace both of those feelings. Later in the book I will be sharing tools to help with the challenges your mind will be throwing at you as you step onto your mat for a full practice, and to help you get there in the first place, but for now just remind yourself that you are your own best teacher and your self-practice is wonderful exactly as it is.

be brave, just try

These next two
tools are about
combining a series of
smaller flows knitted
together to make a
practice.

One that maximises
the time you have
available and
gives you as much
structure or as much
freedom as you need
to make that practice
happen.

Tool #9:

The Wave Practice

Tool #10:

The Mini Practice

9

The Wave Practice

This is the approach to pick when you want your self-practice to reflect the holistic nature of a traditionally sequenced Vinyasa class:

Incorporating the four or five segments that a class would touch upon, one flowing naturally after the other.

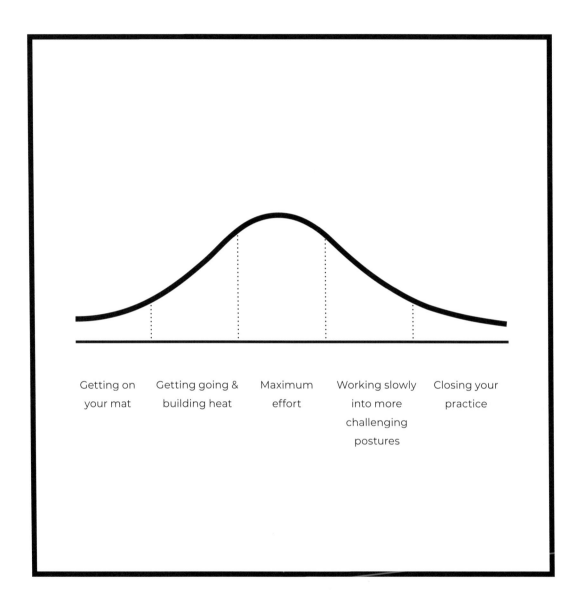

Getting on your mat

Getting going & building heat

Maximum effort

Working slowly into more challenging postures

Closing your practice

In yoga teacher speak,
'the wave' looks like this:

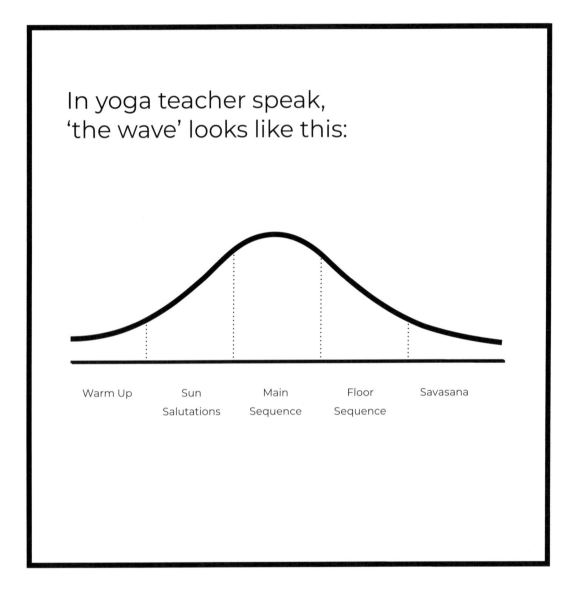

Warm Up　　Sun　　　Main　　　Floor　　Savasana
　　　　Salutations　Sequence　Sequence

This is an extremely effective way of practicing because you are naturally preparing your body for the harder physical work of peak poses or a main sequence.

Using that heat and mind–body connection to work on the deeper postures that the floor sequence often brings, and then winding down towards the harder mental work that is Savasana.

This is also the approach to pick if you crave **structure**.

Getting on your mat by yourself can be scary: not knowing what is meant to come next, or whether you are doing things in the 'right' order. Adding a wave structure to your practice gives you some guidance.

There are no rules though. In fact, with time and with practice, you can and will morph this framework to look wildly different while still adhering to the ethos of this style of practice. But for now, following the pattern and the broad timings can be extremely helpful.

Timings

These are **suggestions** for how to split the time you have available between the different segments.

Some days you might want to leap straight into your Sun Salutations. Other days you might be craving lots of deep hip-opening work and want to expand your floor section to be the majority of your practice. That is completely fine; these timings are just a guide to help you get going.

The Wave Practice Timing Guide

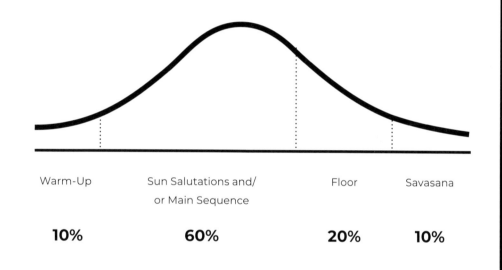

Warm-Up	Sun Salutations and/ or Main Sequence	Floor	Savasana
10%	**60%**	**20%**	**10%**

The following table expands on what these timings could look like for practices lasting from 30 minutes to 120 minutes.

You'll notice the minutes don't always perfectly fit the percentages: they are there to be broad guidelines, not strict rules.

Not least of all because working your

way through a practice with an eye on the clock is unlikely to be enjoyable.

You can check out Tool #4 for help on how to build a playlist that can act as a signal to you during your practice that things are ramping up or cooling down.

Otherwise, simply make a mental note before you start your practice of **roughly** when you want to be moving onto the next part. Remember that this is a tool to **help**, not to hinder: it does not matter one tiny little bit if you stick to these timings!

The Wave Timings Table

		30min.	45min.	60min.	90min.	120min.
Warm Up	10%	3	4	5	10	12
Sun Salutations	20–30%	10	12	10	15	20
Main Sequence(s)	30–40%	10	15	25	35	50
Floor Sequence	20%	5	10	15	20	25
Savasana	10%	3	4	5	10	12

In the table above, I've done the maths bit for you. Very roughly, of course, but enough to get you on your way.

For slightly shorter practices, splitting time more equally between Sun Salutations and your main sequence works well. Have less than 30 minutes? Then Tool #11 The Mini Practice is here for you.

For longer practices, the timings shift towards a longer main sequence. As doing endless Sun Salutations isn't likely to be what you came to your mat for. But as ever, if it is, sun sal your heart out of course!

Sections: **The Wave Practice**

Let's take a closer look at what each of these sections can include, and how you can use different tools from this book for ideas and inspiration at every stage.

1. Warm up

This is all about getting your body ready for what is coming later.

On some days you may know what that is going to be, on other days you might not. So here are a few different approaches that work in each instance:

If in doubt, just move in a way that feels good. It doesn't have to be between actual postures, or with perfect alignment (if that even exists).

I know where my practice is going

Key Body Parts:

Perhaps you have picked something from Tool #1 The Pose Selector as the theme for your practice. Ask yourself this question: what needs a bit of attention before I really start to put weight and effort into it? The classic candidates are going to be things like wrists, shoulders, upper back, hips, hamstrings, feet/ankles.

Opposites:

You know you are going to have a practice focused on one type of posture or one part of your body. Why not spend the few short minutes of your warm up getting into the parts of yourself or your practice which WILL NOT be covered in that main section?

Maybe you are going to have a really flowy creative practice, so start with a long hold headstand to balance that out? Or that backbend practice could start with some gentle forward folds?

I don't know where my practice is going

The Magic Three:

All of us have parts of our bodies that need some extra TLC before we get moving. Getting to know which parts of your body this applies to, and then spending your warm up focused on these, is a great use of time.

Work out what your three are and focus on these in your warm up.

Tuning In:

We touched on this in Tool #5 . Using your warm up as a physical way of tuning in can really set you up to have exactly the practice you need on this particular day. You can do this in lots of ways: moving totally freely and seeing what feedback returns, cycling through simple Downward Facing Dogs to Child poses, or performing a mental or physical body scan – moving each part of your body or directing your mind to it in order to see how it feels.

2. Sun Salutations

Does what it says on the tin.

Perhaps you keep it all traditional, with five Sun Salutation As and five Sun Salutation Bs before moving on. Maybe you do a couple traditional, then start to hack them as per Tool #6. Or, you could go straight to your hacked versions.

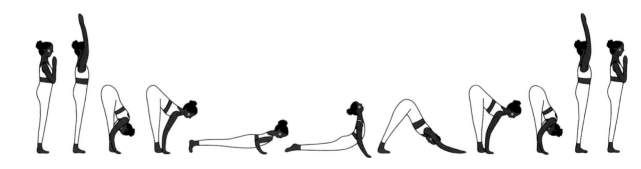

3. Main Sequence

This is where you can get really creative, if that is what will bring you the most joy in your practice.

Use Tool #7 Change It Up and Tool #8 Creative Flows to spice things up and start to link postures in new ways, particularly those you have touched upon in your warm-up and hacked Sun Salutations. If this part of the practice is what scares you most, don't panic. Here are a few tips:

1. Focus on traditional Sun Salutations in the previous section, and then work here on hacking them repeatedly until you get the confidence to start branching out.

2. Remember that uncertainty – feeling awkward, stopping and not knowing what to do next, or not doing the exact same thing on your second side – is natural. Overcoming this is exactly WHY you are practicing yoga (we are going to talk more about this in Tool #11).

3. This is perfect place to integrate something from Tool #2 The Idea Generator and focus on Tools #7 and #8, Change It Up and Creative Flows.

4. Floor Sequence

This is the order I would suggest for the floor section of your practice:

1. **Inversions/arm-balances/drills**

2. **Backbends**

3. **Hips**

4. **Forward Folds**

5. **Twists**

The floor sequence doesn't have to be floor-based posture, but these categories of posture do tend to lend themselves to this part of the practice.

You can do one pose per category, three per category, skip one or two out entirely, or heavily weight towards a category or two. Again, all options are available to you. The limit is your creativity.

But the ORDERING of these categories has a lot of logic behind it, so I would encourage you to follow this.

1. **Inversions / arm-balances / drills:** you are now hopefully both really warm and really connected with your body. So now is the perfect time to focus on trickier postures like inversions and arm-balances, and/or to do drills like core work if you are one of those people that enjoy these things. If not, then move straight along to …

2. **Backbends:** these require a lot of energy and a lot of willpower for most of us at least. Hence placing them towards the beginning of this section when you still have the maximum amount available to you.

   The classic option is to just do three wheel poses, with an appropriate rest in between. Though, of course, the options are much more varied than that (remember, Tool #1 is there to help with this).

3. **Hips:** this is to encourage you to break up the extension of backbends and the flexion of forward folds with postures that allow your spine, and particularly the fluid in your spinal discs, to reset.

4. **Forward Folds:** cooling, calming and closing-in, forward folds are a fantastic penultimate step in your active practice.

5. **Twists:** a very easy category of postures to forget about, but one that will counter those forward folds excellently, while giving your body some final but still hugely beneficial movements.

Lastly, let me end with a request to be kind to yourself. You may have just started to get comfortable with flowing, as perfectly imperfect as that may be, but you have permission to let it go at this stage of your practice. These categories of posture lend themselves towards longer holds and more repetition, and therefore are less easy to connect to one another.

The Ashtanga method of yoga has constructed a way to get around this problem: jump-throughs and jump-backs, so you can of course borrow this for your practice.

Please don't feel like you are doing anything wrong if you simply move from one posture to the next without a pretty or perfect flow in between.

Modify the posture, modify the time,

5. Savasana

We close this section as we should a practice: with Savasana. It is incredibly easy to skip Savasana in a self-practice. What comes next will hopefully persuade you not to.

Savasana is a few quiet moments to acknowledge whatever your mind and body has just done. Then to let that go.

Physically letting go of every part of the body into the floor enables your mind and spirit to let go of the positive or negative connotations of what you just did in your practice. And that in turn is a skill you can learn to take off the mat and into the rest of your life.

This is one of the key features that makes a yoga practice a YOGA practice, and not just an exercise class. Yet, so many of us will come up with excuses not to do it.

This is the compromise I would encourage you to make: **a modified Savasana is better than no Savasana at all.**

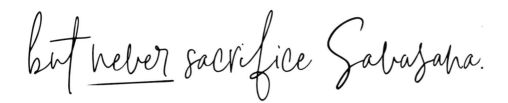

but never sacrifice Savasana.

If your mind will only be quietened on this day, in this practice, by 'doing something', then do something! Take a slightly more active posture. 'Slightly' is a conscious choice of words: this is not a time to be working. But sitting-up, or laying-down in a less exposed shape may be much more calming to you today. That's ok. There are some suggestions on the next pages if this speaks to you.

With time and with practice, it will become easier to transition from a hard day or an intense practice, to a full and long Savasana in the traditional posture.

But if the choice is a modified Savasana or no Savasana at all, then please, please, please pick a modified one.

Make your Savasana work for you: promise yourself you will always do it, even if the form and length changes radically from practice to practice.

Just remember to keep checking in with yourself if you find yourself always leaning towards a short or active Savasana: **there is a reason it is known as the hardest posture of all.**

Savasana suggestions

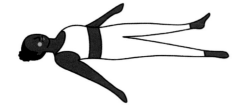 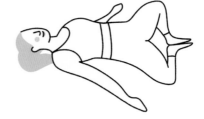

Traditional Savasana
Corpse Pose:

What: Fully reclined on the floor, legs and arms totally relaxed, fully away from the body

When: Great for longer Savasanas as this pose enables full and total relaxation and thus the ability to let the practice and all the thoughts, feelings and beliefs it brought up, go.

Supta Baddha Konasana
Reclined Bound Angle Pose:

What: Reclined, with the soles of the feet together, knees relaxed out. Hands either placed on the body (traditionally one on the heart and one on the belly) or relaxed to the sides, away from the body.

When: A fully reclined and released Savasana can be a lot to ask after shorter or more intense practices, or when you are feeling more tightly wound. This is a great alternative: a more compact pose with body parts touching tends to be more soothing when we aren't fully ready for a total switch-off relaxation.

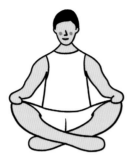

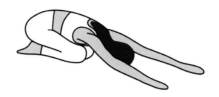

Sukhasana
Easy Pose or
Cross-Legged Pose:

What: Sitting up, legs gently and easily crossed. Hands resting on knees, in the lap, or perhaps pressed together at the heart.

When: Perfect for those super short Savasanas. A few breaths and then off you run.

Balasana
Child's Pose:

What: Arms forwards or back, knees together or wide apart, with or without blocks or blankets or a bolster to give parts of your body the support they may need. Choose what suits you.

When: This option works so well when you are distracted or on edge. Closing the body in entirely, the eyes will almost always naturally close and you can find real rest.

#10

The Mini Practice

Short on time? Or short on energy? A practice does not have to look like a class. This is the tool to prove that.

Not every practice can or should be an hour or more. You can also make the most of smaller pockets of time. Years of conditioning may have taught you about what constitutes a 'real' or 'proper' practice. But even 5 minutes is valuable time on your mat.

Coming immediately after a big section about The Wave Practice, you might think that this format should just be truncated to fit the time available. The message of this tool is that you will make more out of your time by asking yourself to do less.

A mini practice works FANTASTICALLY with just three components:

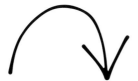

Centre In   Main Practice   Centre Out

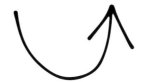

These three simple components give you the maximum permission to flex to whatever it is you are being called to do today.

Note the change in language: 'Warm-Up' becomes 'Centre In' and 'Savasana' becomes 'Centre Out'. It is going to be hard to have a 'full' warm-up if your entire practice is only 5 minutes, or totally let go in Savasana when you only have 30 seconds to allocate to it at the end of a 15-minute flurry of Sun Salutations. THIS IS PERFECTLY OK!

Below there are three different options where a mini practice works well, along with examples of what those mini practices might look like when following the Centre In – Main Practice – Centre Out structure.

Remember, as ever, these are TOOLS not RULES. If these ideas HELP you, then use them. If not, then move right along.

Option 1:
5 minutes

Short and sweet and INSANELY effective for getting your self-practice happening CONSISTENTLY.

If you need some convincing that a 5-minute practice is really worth it, then Tool #13 Lower the Bar is going to be your friend. Or you can try a 5-minute Downward Dog right now and then tell me whether that wasn't some of the hardest physical and mental work you have done in a long time!

Here are a couple of examples:

Long Hold Headstand Mini Practice

 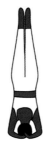 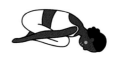

Centre In

Taking three
deep breaths

Main Practice

Four-minute
headstand

Centre Out

One minute
in Child's

Backbend Mini Practice

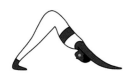 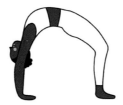 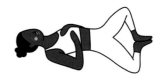

Centre In

20-second holds in an active
Child's and Downward Dog,
three times (two minutes)

Main Practice

Two minutes
of spine rolls and
two 30 second holds
in wheel

Centre Out

Three deep breaths
in Reclined Bound Angle

Option 2: Combining with led classes

The mini practice approach works really well when you are combining a self-practice with regular led (online or in person) classes.

Perhaps the classes you take are all very dynamic and explosive, meaning your mini practices could instead focus on cooler, calmer long-hold work.

Or you made it to a Yin class yesterday and now you want to work up a bit of a sweat.

Pigeon Mini Practice

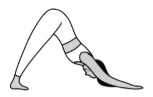 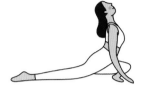 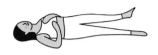

Centre In

One wiggly
Downward Dog
(30 seconds)

Main Practice

Three Legged Dog and five
minute hold in Pigeon on
both sides (11 minutes)

Centre Out

One wiggly Downward Dog
and 10 breaths in Savasana
(one minute)

Sun Sal Mini Practice

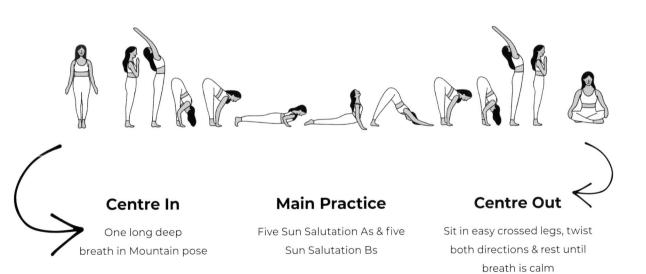

Centre In

One long deep
breath in Mountain pose

Main Practice

Five Sun Salutation As & five
Sun Salutation Bs

Centre Out

Sit in easy crossed legs, twist
both directions & rest until
breath is calm

Option 3: Peak Pose focus

We all have postures we are working towards in our yoga practice (even though we know it's about the practice and not the pose of course). But hey, mastering challenging poses is FUN!

A mini-practice is a PERFECT time to work on these.

Use the skills you learned in Tool #1 The Pose Selector about breaking poses down into their component parts here.

Pincha Mini Practice

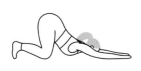
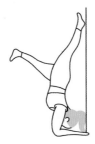
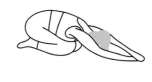

Centre In

Shoulder opening: alternating
between Puppy and
Downward Dog
(one song length)

Main Practice

Shoulder & core strength: Holds
in Dolphin & Forearm Plank
(one song) : Pincha kick-ups
and hold with a wall
(two songs)

Centre Out

Rest in Child's
(one song)

Downward Facing Dog Mini Practice

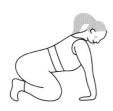
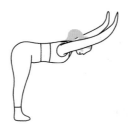
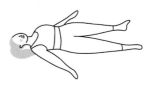

Centre In

Wrist warm-up for
10 breaths

Main Practice

Ragdoll holds, slowly
straightening knees. Shoulder
opening using a wall. 5 minute
hold in Downward Facing Dog
—

Centre Out

Deep breaths in Savasana until
breath is steady and calm

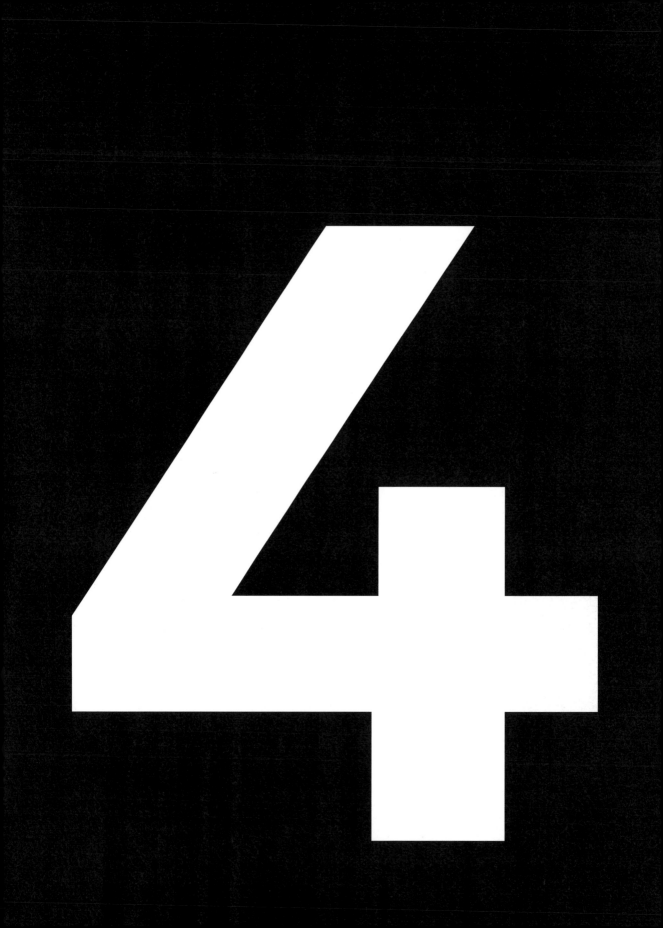

Staying
on Your Mat

"

The very heart of yoga
practice is 'abyhasa'
– steady effort in the
direction you want to go.

-

Sally Kempton

"

The
WHY

Why Is Self-Practice Important for Me?

Understanding the reasons behind your desire and commitment to a yoga self-practice will help you through the tough times when you are unsure, uninspired, and generally un-everything …

There are two tools here to help you with finding your **why**.

One that will always remind you that **the journey is what is valuable**.

And one that will help your steer that journey along **a healthy, sustainable, and personal path**.

Tool #11:

The Mantra

Tool #12:

What Is Your Why?

11

The Mantra

**This is
The Yoga Self-
Practice Mantra.**

It is here for you to use when you are doubting your ability to practice yoga independently.

**Repeat it.
Remember it.
Believe it.**

Self-Practice,
Not Self-Perfection

Self-Practice,
Not Self-Perfection

Self-Practice,
Not Self-Perfection

Self-Practice,
Not Self-Perfection

Self-Practice,
Not Self-Perfection

Self-Practice,
Not Self-Perfection

I want you to read this mantra out loud three times.

Don't want to?

Because it feels weird? Because the people around you will wonder what you are doing? Because you don't want to feel uncomfortable? **That's exactly the point.**

This is just a little reminder of the real challenge we face when starting our self-practice journeys. Feeling uncomfortable – with doing something new, with not being perfect at it, with what people will think of us – is the hurdle.

As you repeat this mantra in your head right now, and again and again when you are on your mat and having a crisis of confidence, remember that THIS is the yoga you are practicing too.

You need to get comfortable with the voice inside you that says you can't do it. The one that tells you to stop. The one that criticises, nit-picks and cuts you down.

Just as you practice feeling physically challenged in a tricky pose, you also practice feeling mentally challenged.

This mantra will help you. Repeat it every time you need it. It's an essential tool of your yoga self-practice.

Self-Practice, Not
Perfection. **Self-Pr**
ce, Not Self-Perfec
Self-Practice, Not
Perfection. **Self-Pra**
ce, Not Self-Perfec
Self-Practice, Not
Perfection. **Self-Pra**
ce, Not Self-Perfec
Self-Practice, Not
Perfection. **Self-Pra**

elf-Perfection. **Sel**

ctice, Not Self-Per

:ion. **Self-Practice**

Self-Perfection. **Sel**

ctice, Not Self-Per

:ion. **Self-Practice**

Self-Perfection. **Sel**

ctice, Not Self-Per

:ion. **Self-Practice,**

Self-Perfection. **Sel**

ctice, Not Self-Per

#12

—

What Is Your Why?

Find the purpose behind your yoga practice. And make that purpose work FOR you, rather than against you.

The clearer you are on what the WHY is behind your yoga practice, the easier it is going to be to do the work necessary to achieve your goals.

You clearly have something that is driving you to delve into the world of yoga practice, especially a self-practice.

And let's be honest, it is going to be work. Enjoyable work hopefully, but it will require effort, dedication, consistency, and some sweat. Maybe even some tears.

Finding your why will also help answer some of the harder questions that are likely to pop up as you continue your yoga journey.

If you know what your ultimate driver is, then it's much easier to answer these questions in the most rational way possible.

Finding Your Why

What is the big, juicy, overall driving reason that you practice yoga? Why are you here? **This is your self-practice goal.**

Self-Practice Goals:

If you took one look at that box and skipped right ahead, I don't blame you. It's a scary question to answer!

Go on, head back up there and see if you can fill something in … we will come back to this a little later.

Remember, this will hopefully be something that changes over the many months, and years, of your yoga practice. Don't feel like what you write today has to be true forever. Here are some prompts which may help:

Physical:

Do you want to improve your fitness or flexibility, or recover from injury?

Well-being:

Do you want to create calm or do more of something that makes you happy?

Spiritual:

Do you want to connect with yourself or tap into something more powerful?

Achieving your self-practice goal will require substantial and sustained focus over a long period of time.

Rather than trying to bite off the whole thing in every practice, I would really recommend that you set yourself weekly or monthly focused goals that will help you reach your self-practice goal.

These goals will be much more effective if they give you **A KISS**.

Achievable

Kind

In Control

Specific

Sustainable

Achievable

Any goal setting exercise works best if it's full of manageable things you can do to move step by step towards the overall objective.

Please don't be too ambitious to start with. It's easy to get super excited at the start of any new project and take too much on. This is a recipe for feeling rubbish about yourself when you realise you can't achieve what you set out to.

Having goals that are too ambitious can make us LESS likely to do the work needed to achieve them.

 Set yourself up for success with an achievable target.

For example, just one more time on your mat or class per week. If you find it too easy that's fine; you can always stretch the target next month.

Kind

Is your goal and the way you are approaching it something you would want your very favourite person in the whole world to set for themselves?

If not, maybe you could be a little kinder to yourself.

5 minutes is enough. One Downward Dog is enough. One class is enough. (We are going to talk more about this in the next tool).

YOU ARE ALREADY ENOUGH, JUST AS YOU ARE.

Let's say that again …

YOU ARE ALREADY ENOUGH, JUST AS YOU ARE.

It Is wonderful to wish for and to work towards more of course. But you ARE ENOUGH.

Set yourself some goals that you'll enjoy working towards. A basic fact of the human condition is that we are all more likely to repeatedly do things we enjoy!

In Control

You can't meet your goals without making them work for you rather than against you.

Instead of focusing on what you can't control – the outcome – focus on what you can control – your commitment to the practice.

You might want six pack abs but what if you have a body that won't show a visible six pack? You might want to become a yoga teacher but what if your local studio doesn't have space for a new teacher or a time slot that works for you?

Even goals like 'touch my toes' or 'hold a headstand in the middle of the room' may still be out of reach no matter how hard you try.

Instead of being a slave to issues beyond your control, morph these goals into something that serves you:

Outcome Focused Goal becomes Practice Focused Goal

o 'Develop six pack abs' becomes 'add one core strength drill to every practice'.
o 'Become a yoga teacher' becomes 'sign up for yoga teacher training'
o 'Practice every day' becomes 'make a conscious decision daily about whether a physical yoga practice will serve your self-practice goal'.

Sustainable

The journey is long, and it will require patience. Change comes, but only if you keep showing up consistently over time.

The journey is long, and it will require patience. Change comes, but only if you keep showing up consistently over time.

The biggest challenge most people face when it comes to yoga is sticking with it. You might meet your goals in week one but are you going to be able to keep it up indefinitely? Or was it the energy of having something new to focus on that got you through?

Choose goals that you really want to work towards and that will tempt you onto your mat.

Specific

If your weekly and monthly goals are going to be effective, then they need to be specific.

It's all well and good to say that you want to 'get good at yoga', 'become really flexible and strong', or 'learn to control my emotions' but how will you measure your progress against these?

Instead, here are four approaches to setting specific yoga practice goals. Notice that your self-practice can just be one component of these.

1. **'Just Get on My Mat':**

o It doesn't matter whether it's one Downward Facing Dog while dinner is cooking, a 90-minute class at a local studio, or something in between. This approach gives you the freedom and support to see yoga as something that is meant to look different depending on how you are feeling or what else is going on in your life.

o Pick a target: once, twice, four, seven times a week.

2. 'I Need to Build a Foundation':

o Great if you are still at the beginning of your journey.

o Perhaps you need to take more classes to help you develop a solid understanding of the postures and your own practice. Or you need to build your confidence to self-practice so want to try three Sun Salutations by yourself at home three times a week.

3. 'Try Something New':

o Perfect if you are stuck in a bit of a yoga rut.

o Always going to the same classes, doing the same thing when you step on your mat, or too nervous to try a particular pose or type of yoga? This one might be for you.

o First, work out exactly what your rut is and WHY you are stuck there. This may require some serious self-reflection. See if you can do three to five levels of asking why. For example, don't just ask yourself, 'why do I only go to this type of class?'. Take that answer and ask why again. And so on.

o Your target could be to try one new class of a different style of yoga every other week, or to attend three workshops over the next six months focused on a specific area, or to try a different one of the tools in this book every week in your self-practice.

4. 'A Little Bit of Everything':

o All of these appeal?! Pick and mix! Create something that works for you.

Self-Practice Goals:

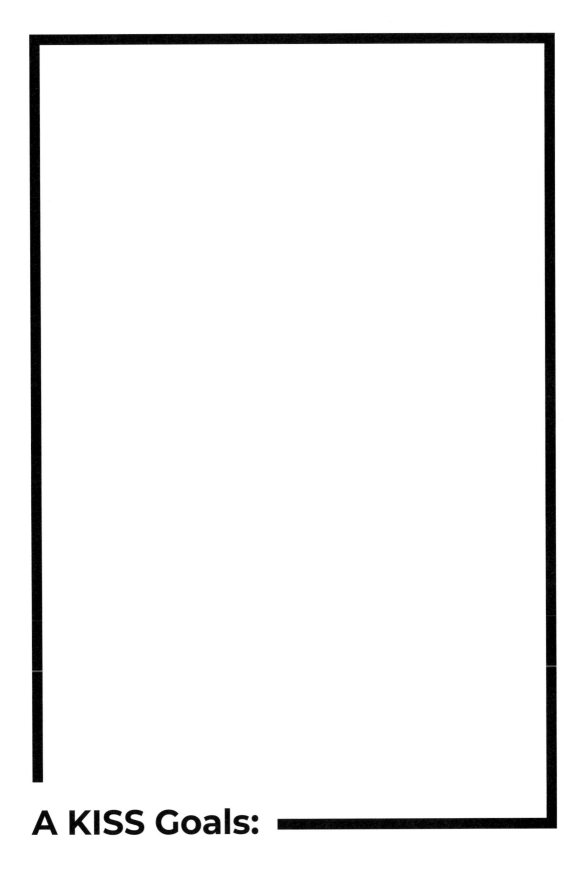

A KISS Goals:

The
WHERE
& WHEN

How Do I Make a Self-Practice Actually Happen?

This is where we get super practical:

Knowing what or how to do a self-practice means nothing unless you actually get on your mat!

The next three
tools will help you
find your **where**
and your **when**.

The time and the
space you need
to make self-
practice a part
of your life.

Consistently,
and over the
long-term.

Tool #13:

Lower the Bar

Tool #14:

Make Your Mat Your Mate

Tool #15:

Finding the Time

Finding the time and space
for your practice
can be hard.

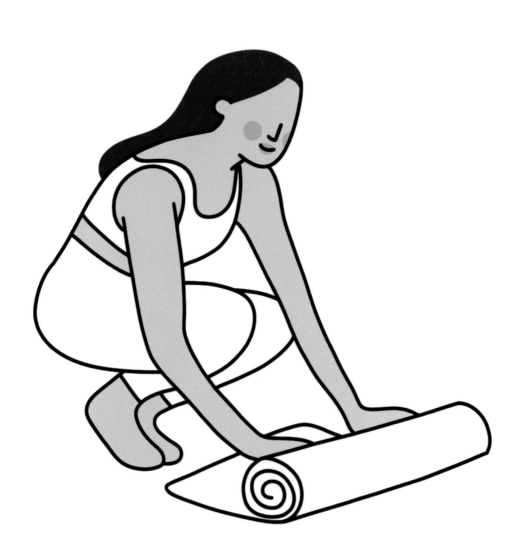

Because lofty goals, and fun flows, and juicy postures are all great. Really great.

But if it was easy to get this stuff done, everyone would be doing it, wouldn't they?

We all live incredibly busy and intense lives. Being connected to work 24-7, nurturing the love of our family and friends, the FOMO that a life lived with social media creates ... all of these are big asks. Put them together, and maybe add running a household, or studying, or dealing with illness or injury, and you won't have much spare time, forget about spare mental capacity. These tools are here to help.

#13
—

Lower the Bar

Change comes only through consistency, whatever your goal may be.

Take one look at any yoga studio schedule and it's easy to get the message that a 'proper' practice is 45 to 75 minutes long, if not more. But if the bar to getting on your mat is that you need 45 minutes for a practice to 'count', then you are going to have far fewer practices.

You absolutely must, must, **must** disabuse yourself of this point of view.

It is not just wrong, it will also likely be one of the highest hurdles to your self-practice, so lower the bar.

Have you ever held a Downward Dog or a headstand for 3 minutes? That is hard work! What about taking a moment in a busy day, interlacing your hands behind your back and lifting them up to open your chest as you take a deep breath? Try it and tell me if you don't instantly feel the benefits.

Small amounts of time, movement and effort can have a HUGE impact: in the moment that you do them, and especially as you repeat them again and again over days, months and years.

It's much more manageable and realistic to think about 5 or 10 minutes on your mat.

With luck and kindness many of your practices will become much longer than a single pose or a handful of minutes, but only if you start.

So, **lower the bar**. Truly start believing that:

One pose is a practice,
5 minutes is a practice.
Any practice is a proper practice.

14

Make Your Mat Your Mate

Here are another two deceptively simple steps to help you lower the hurdle to practice.

Get a mat you love

The right amount of sticky, comfy, pretty, spacious, portable ... whatever it is that YOU need for YOUR practice, and that works for YOUR budget.

You're hopefully going to be spending a lot of time on it. Make it special.

Truly, you do not need fancy designer yoga leggings or whizz-bang props to help in your self-practice journey, but an investment in a yoga mat that stops you slip-sliding, helps you find the right alignment, and that tempts you to get onto it, is worth every penny that is realistic for you to allocate to it.

Make your mat accessible

Keep your mat rolled out where you can see it. Or if you don't have enough space to do so, keep it out of its case and in your eye line.

You'll notice that I said deceptively simple in the introduction to this tool. This part of Tool #14 sounds so incremental that you will probably be inclined to skip right over it: surely something so small cannot make that big a difference?!

Seeing your mat multiple times a day, being able to step onto it with minimal effort WILL make you get onto it, and practice on it, more often.

Seriously. The impact of something so simple may make you question your own sanity, so apologies in advance!

Maybe just one Downward Dog while the kettle boils, perhaps a 10-minute hip-opening sequence before dinner, or even one Sunday afternoon that two-hour practice that once seemed impossible to do by yourself.

15

Finding
the Time

What good is the ability and the will to self-practice unless you actually find the time in your life for it? Use this tool to make it happen.

Start off by assessing your current approach. You might find you already have different approaches to different parts of your practice. Or that the rules you find work in other parts of your life, like your career, you have never thought to apply to your self-practice.

On the next page, I lay out the three different approaches to scheduling your yoga practice. Spelling out this spectrum is all about making you conscious that there are other approaches you can turn to when the one you have been using most is not working so well anymore. Which happens to all of us.

Switching things up with your scheduling, or lack there of, can be a really useful way to get more practice into your life.

Also think about how you can mix and match these approaches for the various parts of your practice. Classes might need a different plan to self-practice. Getting on your mat to practice inversions might come more easily than doing the same for backbends.

Super organised, prefer to go with the flow, or somewhere in between?

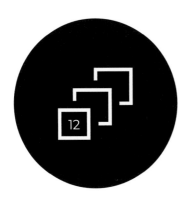

Diarise

Doesn't happen if you don't put it in your diary? Then start adding your yoga time in.

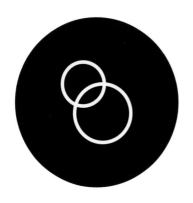

Combine

Try blocking out a few slots a week for a self-practice and then add in mini-practices when the opportunity strikes.

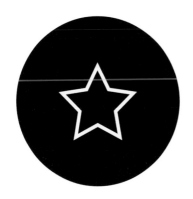

Be Spontaneous

Want to prioritise respecting what your body rather than the clock is telling you? Then this is the option for you.

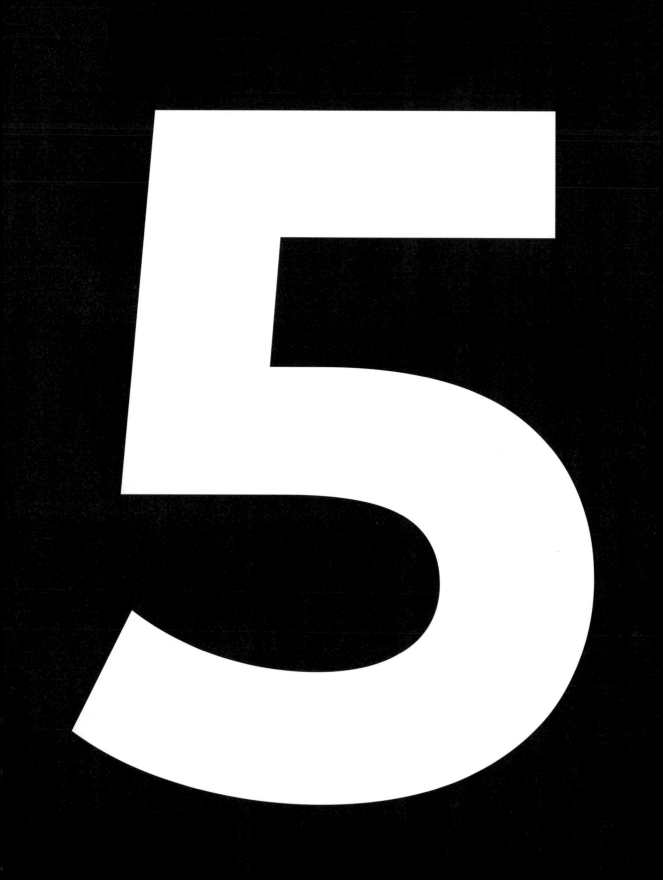

Progressing
on Your Mat

"

You don't practice yoga
to get better at yoga.

You practice yoga
to get better at LIVING.

-

Unknown

"

The
WHAT
NEXT

How Do I Ensure Progression While Self-Practicing?

What is progress in yoga?

Is it getting to the more advanced poses, practicing more often, for longer, or something else?

These five tools will
help you find your own
personal path to progress.

Progress may look very
different to you than it
does for others.

And this is exactly why it is
so important to spend the
time working out what this
looks like FOR YOU.

Tool #16:

Press Record

Tool #17:

The Debrief

Tool #18:

Journalling

Tool #19:

Build Your Village

Tool #20:

The Learning Triad

#16

—

Press Record

Here we get you over one of the biggest hurdles of a yoga self-practice: the fear of doing it wrong.

This tool is an instruction to film your practice and watch it back.

The fear of doing postures 'wrong' while self-practicing alone is real, and totally legitimate. While I am an advocate of the view that there is really no objective 'wrong', just what is wrong for your body as it is today, that doesn't mean that we couldn't all benefit from refining the alignment in our practices and making sure we are using the muscles and movements we think we are.

This is where videoing your practice comes in.

I will stop right here
and say clearly: no-
one apart from you
ever needs to see
these videos.

You do not have
to post them
to Instagram.

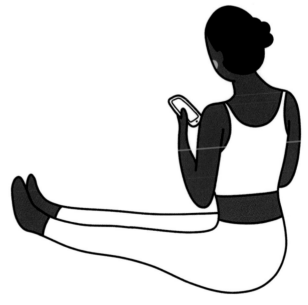

But do record yourself, either regularly or every once in a while, **for two reasons:**

Brain and Body
Disconnections

What we think we are doing with our bodies and what we are actually doing with them can be very different things (watch the vast majority of people on the dancefloor at a wedding for evidence of this!).

You can be in what feels like an incredibly deep backbend, yet a picture could show that all of the bend is in your lower back, with none in your upper back. Or a glance in the mirror could show a hunched-up reflection in a forward fold, rather than that nice flat back you imagine.

Or maybe you are hypermobile and think you are not dumping into a vulnerable joint, but when a teacher asks you to brace, you can see the big change that brings.

Watching yourself back on video will help you spot all these tweaks, and more.

Brain and Body
Connections

Most of us will struggle with executing with our own bodies the image we see in our heads, on our teachers or on our screens. However, the vast majority of us are pretty darn good at recognising in a pose that we can SEE what can be tweaked, adjusted, optimised or improved.

When you have the foundation you need for a yoga self-practice (see Part 2 for help with this), and are working to keep learning (which is what Tool #20 is for), you WILL have a reasonable sense of what is a good, a better, or a BEST FOR YOU version of a posture WHEN YOU CAN SEE YOURSELF DOING THAT POSTURE.

This is why videoing your practice is so powerful. It might not be as magical as having an amazing teacher watching you and cueing those tweaks in real time. But in one very important way it is even more powerful than that: because you will be working it out for yourself. The lessons we learn ourselves stick so much better than ones others teach us.

Still not quite sure whether your eye will be good enough to spot where you can tweak? Watch some other people's flows on Instagram, or in a class, particularly people at your level or newer to the practice. You might just surprise yourself.

Top Tips for Recording Your Practice

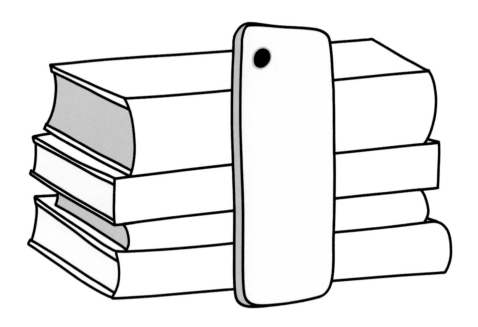

No need to buy a fancy phone stand – these options will all work just as well

o A few well-placed books.

o Wedging your phone in a large cup with a sock.

o Propping your phone up on the skirting board.

Watch yourself back at speed

o Using apps: check out www.yoga-self-practice.com/blog for our favourites.

o Manually: press pause on the playback on your phone and scroll forwards through the video at your own speedy pace. That way you can easily stop and watch any bits that look particularly excellent (or strange!).

Not enough space on your phone? This one is for iPhone users but I am sure the other brands have something similar

o Enable iCloud Photo Library. Go to Settings -> Photos & Camera -> Turn ON the option for iCloud Photo Library AND the option to Optimise iPhone Storage.

o This means older photos/videos will be saved to the cloud (you might need to buy more storage space).

o You can still see them in your photo library but to watch the full video or see the high-resolution version of the picture, your phone will download it from the Cloud when you open it.

17

The Debrief

Taking a few moments after your practice to reflect on how it went and to explore what that means for future practices is a really valuable use of your time.

So do exactly that: debrief yourself after your practice. Ask yourself how it went, and how it felt.

This tool will help you review your practice in a truly holistic way. We all come to our practice with baggage: from mundanity of to-do lists, to more profound expectations for our postures, bodies, and perhaps even our lives.

The answers you get when you actively debrief yourself after you practice might surprise you. Perhaps that sweaty session that usually charges you up was strangely draining today. Or, with hindsight, your backbends felt a little close to the edge to be safe?

Give yourself the time to ask the question and to hear the response. This can be something you just mentally run through in the few minutes after your practice, or something more formal you write down after every one of your practices.

My Debrief Checklist	

What worked?

What didn't work?

How did it feel?

What was hard?

What came easy?

What might you do differently next time?

What surprised you the most?

#18
—

Journalling

Writing down a quick summary of what your practice entailed, and your thoughts and feelings about it is a wonderful tool to build understanding.

If you regularly both record your practice and debrief, then it is but a hop, skip, and a jump to keeping a yoga journal. The act of putting pen to paper enables your brain to process complex ideas, make new connections and see patterns, trends and pitfalls in our practice.

It's incredibly helpful to be able to look back and see how you felt about a tough Vinyasa class last month, or when you first 'got' a tricky posture, or spot that you always feel exhausted when you push yourself too hard the week before your period.

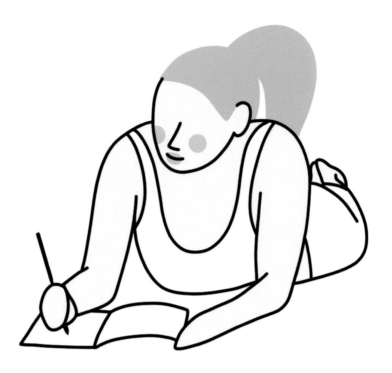

Whether you want to buy a dedicated notebook, set up a few standard prompts to copy/paste in a notes app on your phone, or print out the following templates to create your own book, this can be as formal or as low-key as suits you.

The desire to keep a consistent journal might just be the final push you need to get on to your mat on those days where it's a challenge.

Remember, you can download and/or print blank copies of these templates at www.yoga-self-practice.com.

Here are a few different suggested yoga journal templates that might work for you.

Feel free to 'hack' them to better reflect the questions or prompts that will best serve your practice and journalling experience.

Weekly Journal Template

A free-form template where you can jot down any information about classes you took, books you read, or your self-practice sessions. Great for those that want to be thinking about practicing something more days a week than not.

	Self-Practice		Classes	
Monday				
Tuesday				
Wednesday				
Thursday				
Friday				
Saturday				
Sunday				
Time Spent: Total				

Practice
Journal Template

This one will help to reinforce that every practice counts, no matter how (in) frequently you manage them or what they contain.

Date:		Practice Info	

What I did:

How it felt:

Note to self:

Yoga Prompt
Journal Template

Similar to the Practice Journal Template but with more structure around de-briefing your practice.

Practice Info	

Favourite Pose(s) today:

Hardest Pose(s) today:

What worked, what didn't work:

What was hard, what came easy:

Something to do differently next time:

Something that surprised me in my practice:

19

Build Your Village

It takes a village, right?! Doing this stuff alone isn't easy. This tool will help you identify your yoga village.

This will be your support system along this wonderful yoga journey.

Finding people that share your interest in yoga can help in so many ways: to keep you accountable for showing up to class, to cheer you on when you get stuck in a rut, to answer your questions about mats and leggings and impossible transitions.

All of this might require you to step outside of your comfort zone.

There are many, **many** parts of our yoga practice which require us to do exactly that, so just consider this your yoga for the day!

Trust me when I
say that there are
so many people out
there looking to find
their yoga village
too: you are not the
only one and they
will be so grateful
when you have the
bravery to introduce
yourself and get the
ball rolling.

Your Existing Circle

Is there anyone in your life already into yoga, or who wants to get started? Not sure? ASK!

Tell the people that are important to you that yoga is important to you. You will either get their support, or perhaps find someone who will want to get involved as well. A win-win.

In Class

Does the same person usually attend your regular weekly class? You're allowed to say hi!

Introduce yourself and see if they want a grab a coffee afterwards.

If this feels really challenging, then workshops, or classes like AcroYoga tend to provide a more natural environment to start chatting to people.

Social Media

It's called social for a reason. The yoga community on Instagram especially is one of warmest, most welcoming, uplifting and supportive ones out there.

You just need to find your people.

Search hashtags (pop in #yoga and all sorts will come up), join challenges, like and comment on other people's posts, be brave and direct message those you connect with.

And don't forget, the @yogaselfpractice Instagram community is here for you. I founded it in the summer of 2018 to be a place full of real people of all body types, races, and practice levels, showing up to do their everyday practices in their homes surrounded by kids/pets/mess/real life and all. I would love to see you there. And you can always reach out to me via my personal page @somewhat_rad.

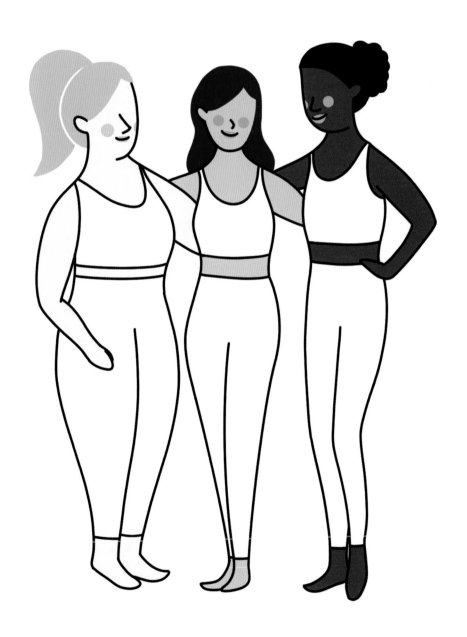

20

The Learning Triad

This might be the last tool in the book but it's also one of the most important.

Use the Learning Triad as a blueprint to guide you forwards to continue learning as much about this practice as you can.

Self-practice is, by its very definition, a journey of learning: about yoga and yourself. You will learn so much about both every single time you step on your mat.

Learning from diverse sources maximises and reinforces that which you learn. This tool will help you take advantage of the entire Learning Triad in yoga.

What the hell is a Learning Triad?! I'm glad you asked!

Learning has three components: being taught, studying, and experience. Each one feeds into the others.

Active Study
Direct Instruction
Your Experience

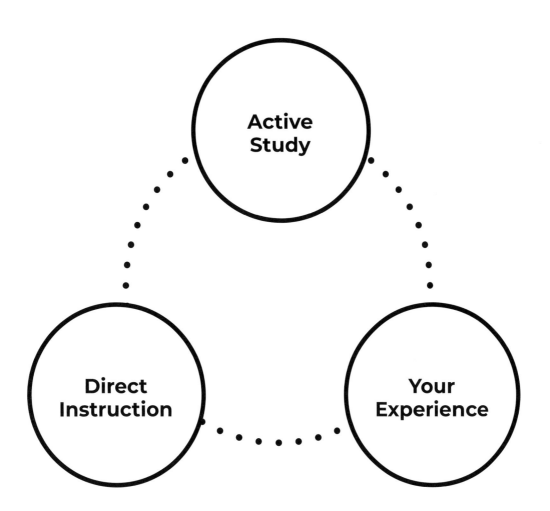

Each one of us has a natural bias towards how we learn best.

Maybe from a teacher in a class, on our own via YouTube videos or books, or simply messing around alone on our mats.

Looking at the triad, ask yourself two key questions:

1. **Are you fully exploring the component you naturally favour?**

2. **Are you making an effort to further explore the other two?**

There are aspects of all our lives that will limit how far this is going to be possible: money, time, location, level of ability or confidence. And that's ok! So please add the addendum 'to the best of my ability and current personal circumstances' to both of these questions.

Just know that when you get stuck in a rut, frustrated, or want to deepen your experience of yoga, this is one of the most effective tools there is. After all:

The more you learn, the more you practice. The more you practicse, the more you learn.

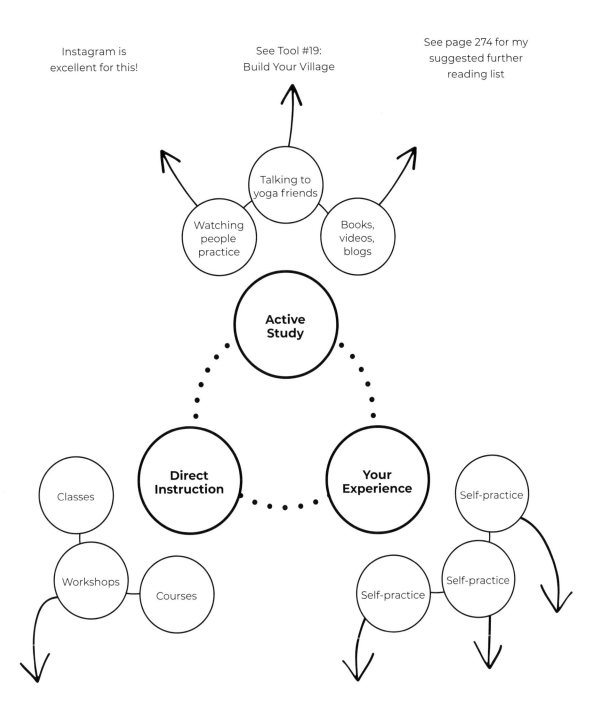

Instagram is excellent for this!

See Tool #19: Build Your Village

See page 274 for my suggested further reading list

Watching people practice

Talking to yoga friends

Books, videos, blogs

Active Study

Direct Instruction

Your Experience

Classes

Workshops

Courses

Self-practice

Self-practice

Self-practice

Workshops provide the most bang for your buck, both in terms of time and money, in my opinion!

Can you spot my bias here?! Studying and being taught are essential learning tools. Only self-practice – due to its very independence – will bring you true experience!

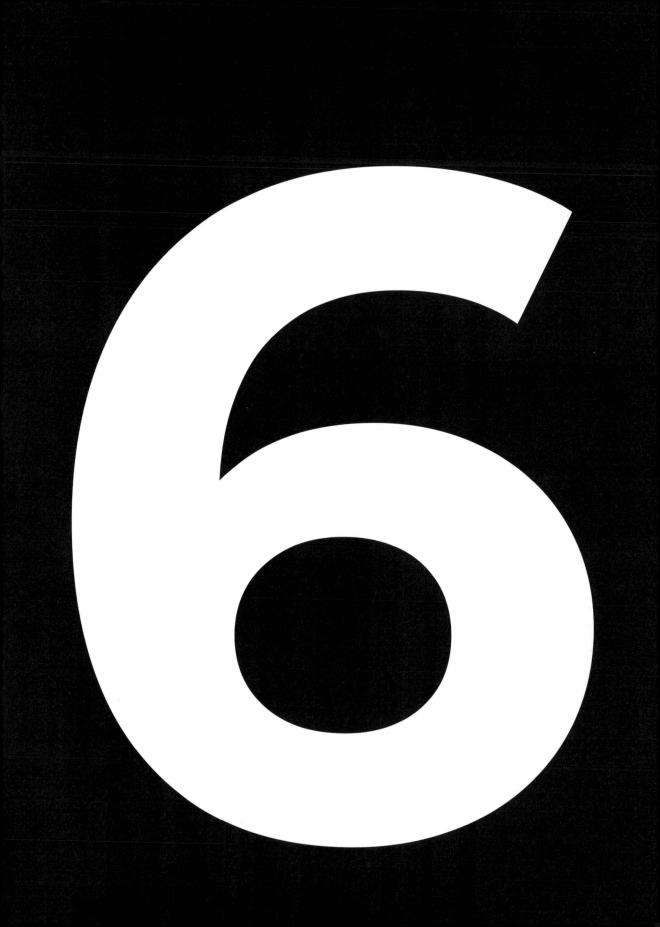

Your Questions Answered

"

For many years I mistook
discipline as ambition.

Now I believe it to be more
about consistency.

Do get on the mat. Practice
and life are not that different.

-

Judith Hanson Lasater

Questions and Answers

This self-practice malarkey isn't easy. If it was, everyone would be doing it!

It is totally natural to have more questions, or for issues to arise as your tread this path. Below are some of the most frequently asked questions and answers.

There are also more resources to help you and where you can ask any questions not covered below.

Instagram: for tips, inspiration and community go to @somewhat_rad and @yogaselfpractice

Website: www.yoga-self-practice.com

With so many types of yoga, teachers, and ways to learn, getting started on your yoga journey can be confusing.

The good news is that EVERY yogi you see doing fancy stuff on Instagram or in your local class was once where you are right now.

Every. Single. One.

What kind of yoga should I do?

To get to where they are, you need to first work out what type of physical yoga, or asana, you want to do and the approach to learning that works best for you. This is about assessing three things:

1. **Your current state of fitness and flexibility**

2. **Your background in sport/ movement/dance**

3. **What you are looking to achieve out of your practice**

The diagram opposite gives a brief introduction to the main different styles of yoga and my take on what the key features of each are.

However, it is always worth remembering that most teachers and studios have a huge amount of leeway over how they teach.

This is particularly so for styles like Vinyasa (which also includes types like Jivamukti and Anasura) and Hatha (which is a broad encompassing style where the focus is on holding individual postures rather than moving between them).

You may well find a Vinyasa teacher who teaches a set sequence, or a Yin teacher who likes to add a bit of flow between postures. Try different ones until you find the right fit.

Creative

Styles without a set sequence:
it's all up to your teacher

Active

Styles where you will
actively hold in the postures

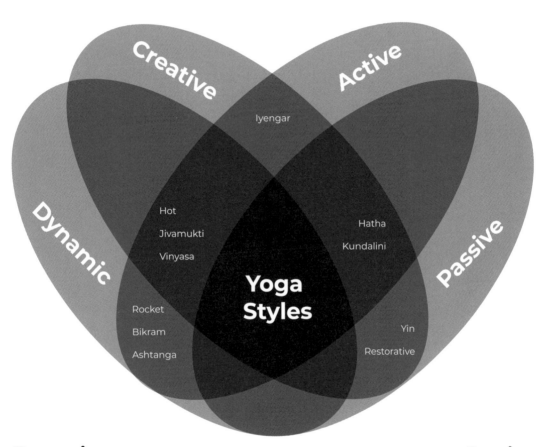

Creative

Active

Iyengar

Dynamic

Hot
Jivamukti
Vinyasa

Hatha
Kundalini

Passive

**Yoga
Styles**

Rocket
Bikram
Ashtanga

Yin
Restorative

Dynamic

Styles where you will move with
pace and likely buld up as sweat

Passive

Styles where you be more
passive in the postures

It's easy to focus on the physical aspects of what you can/can't do and what you want to be able to achieve through starting a yoga practice. But I would really encourage you to think about what kind of experience you enjoy the most.

Change ONLY happens with consistency and you are only going to be able to achieve consistency in this new yoga habit if you ENJOY it.

Some people thrive with the boot-camp style of training and the feeling they have 'punished' a workout. But while yoga is amazing for the strength, fitness and flexibility gains it will bring, this is a mindset that will likely bring lots of injuries – physical and mental – when you are at the start of your yoga journey.

Instead, find a style, a class, a teacher THAT YOU ENJOY. Maybe it's not the most intense version, perhaps you don't burn a million calories, or push your muscles to shaking point. But you will see greater 'results' by turning up again and again over a prolonged period of time than you ever will only making it to a handful classes before you can't face going again because it makes you feel rubbish about yourself.

This is especially true when your ultimate goal is to be able to practice on your own.

How can I best learn?

You need to work out how to balance the trade-offs of modern life – money, time availability, convenience – with how you learn best.

Some of us will do better in a group setting, with the extra motivation that brings. Others would rather go away, quietly read and work things out for themselves.

Some have the luxury of being able to invest both time and money in their practice, while others have other more pressing priorities and need a more economical solution.

The chart opposite lays out the myriad of options available, showing the trade-offs between investment and level of input from a teacher.

Of course, this is all very personal and circumstance dependent, but at a very general level, some investment in an option towards the top right is likely to get to you a place where you can utilise the options in the bottom left both safely and effectively.

Don't forget to head back to the self-practice checklist on page 51 when you think you might be ready to give an independent yoga practice a go.

This chart lays out the myriad of options available, showing the trade-offs between investment and level of input from a teacher.

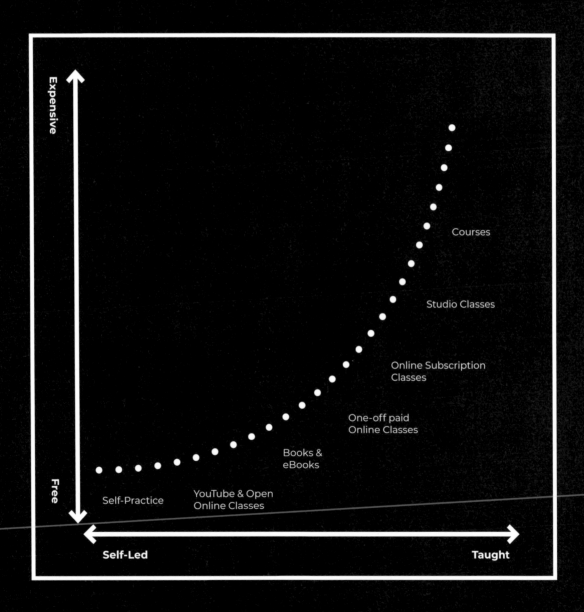

What I am meant to do if I don't know how to do certain poses?

Go out and learn them. Sounds simple, I know, but I also know simple doesn't mean easy! You can study from a book, or learn from a teacher, or go to workshop. There are so many options, you just have to find what works for you.

Then you get to come back to your self-practice and build EXPERIENCE using what you have learned.

Tool #20 The Learning Triad is here to help with all of this.

What if I do the postures wrong?

The yoga police will come and arrest you and you will never be allowed to practice again. Joke!

Let me remind you that there is no objectively 'wrong' way to practice a pose.

There is only what is wrong for your body and what is wrong for your goals. Both of which may change day to day, practice to practice.

The one universal truth for a yoga practice, be it by yourself or with a teacher, is that no-one wants to get injured. If you are worried you are doing certain postures in a way that is going to injure you, then stop. Seek help: ask a teacher in person or online, or take a class or workshop focused on the problem area, or go and see a qualified physiotherapist.

If you are not sure whether you are doing things in the optimal way for your body, then again, seek help or continue to study. Study the posture, study your body. Go carefully. With time, practice and study, you will work it out.

I'm injured. Should I still be practicing?

If you are injured, you should always, ALWAYS visit a medical professional. You have one body and it is precious. Treat it as such.

Once you have an expert opinion, then you can decide about whether to practice. Sometimes the very best yoga you can do is no physical yoga at all. Maybe you finally have the time you need to read that yoga philosophy book?

If you and your medical team decide you can do some form of practice, then work out how you want to modify your practice. One of the most wonderful things about yoga is its flexibility: it may feel like you can't continue a practice while staying off your hands, not using a foot or eliminating backbends, but you can. It will look different to your non-injured practice but that's fine.

If you speak to most experienced yogis, they will tell you that the times they were injured were some of the most valuable learning experiences they've had – both about themselves and their yoga practice. It will be hard and you are allowed to feel rubbish about it. But once you are through to the other side, chances are you will be grateful for what this injury has taught you.

I'm afraid of hurting myself without a teacher there to guide me.

If you are used to taking classes with a teacher, it will feel scary to be without one.

Go carefully, listen to your body, record and review your practices (Tools #16 Press Record, #17 The Debrief,

#18 Journalling), and use smart sequencing (as discussed in Tools #9 The Wave Practice and #10 The Mini Practice) to make sure your body is ready for what you are asking it to do.

What if I forget to do exactly the same thing on both sides?

The yoga police will knock down your door again and rearrest you. (Did I get another smile?!)

Everyone forgets poses or gets them in the wrong order: even the most experienced teachers in classes they've prepared endlessly for.

Accept that this is part of what the practice is about: making mistakes and continuing on. Getting to practice on your mat with small mistakes like this will help you off your mat when the mistakes are bigger.

Here are some practical tips to help with your consistency:

o Go for a simpler flow. It's ok to keep things simple! With time and practice, you will find more complex flows coming more easily and with fewer 'mistakes'. Promise.

- Start on your non-dominant side for a change. This often helps your brain pay more attention to what you are doing and thus better remember it for the second side.

- You are allowed to stop mid-flow. Take a Child's Pose or Downward Dog and either try to remember, or if you have been videoing yourself, use the video to remind yourself.

I get stuck after one or two poses or flows and don't know what to do next.

This is completely normal. It might take you a few weeks or even months for this to stop happening. It can be super frustrating, but just as you wouldn't expect to be able to do a new and difficult pose first time, self-practice is a skill that will improve with time and dedication.

This is also where combining the different tools from this book and planning things out a little before you get on your mat might help. Spend 2 minutes – literally, no more – doing the following:

i. Pick a category for your practice: use Tool #1 The Pose Selector

ii. Pick something from Tool #2 The Idea Generator to make it interesting

iii. Use either Tool #9 The Wave Practice or Tool #10 The Mini Practice to VERY briefly sketch out your timings or sections

iv. Jot all of this it down on a piece of paper you can have at the top of your mat

v. Off you go

Tool #11 The Mantra is also essential on days like this! Tell yourself at the start, and again and again throughout, that it is ok to stop and think about what you want to do next. It is ok for things not to be perfect, smooth, or without doubt. It's ok to feel awkward and annoyed. That is what the practice is for: to teach you to be ok with all those feelings.

Keep going. You've got this!

I get distracted when I practice by myself. Is this normal, and how do I prevent it?

Of course, it is normal. It might even be a blessing in disguise. The more often your mind wanders, the more times you get to practice the Awareness-Focus loop that is a hugely powerful outcome of a yoga practice.

Observe and acknowledge the distractions. If they stop your practice fully, then maybe there are some ways you can reduce them, for example, moving into a different room or practicing at a different time of day. If the distractions simply make you lose concentration, then embrace the opportunity to bring yourself back into focus and carry right on.

It is also totally ok to have to interrupt a practice to answer the door, respond to a family member or take something out of the oven. Remember, if you set the hurdle so high that you will only practice when you can guarantee ZERO distractions, then I bet you will NEVER practice. Tool #13 Lower The Bar is here to help on this one.

Do what you can, when you can. Be proud of what you do manage. It is enough. You are enough.

How do you fit a self-practice in? I'm just so busy!

This is all about lowering the bar (hello Tool #13 Lower the Bar), finding times that work for you (hello Tool #15 Finding the Time) and making it as easy as you can to get on your mat (hello Tool #14 Make Your Mat Your Mate).

A lot of people feel they need to practice in the morning in order to have a 'proper' practice. That's great if mornings work for you but there is nothing wrong with practicing at different times of the day. Find what works for you.

Your practice schedule might also look very different on weekdays vs. weekends, at different times of the year, or different times in your life. That is not only ok: that is EXACTLY what you want it to be. A practice that fits in with your life for the long term is one that keep giving you what you need, even when your needs change radically.

All my self-practice sessions are so short. I just run out of ideas or go too quickly.

First, let go of the idea that a long practice equals a good practice. Maybe you are already doing exactly what your body and mind really need.

However, if you really do want to extend your practices, then Tool #9 The Wave Practice is your friend (as is the playlist builder which is part of Tool #3 Beats). There is no need to stick rigidly to the suggested times but having them as a guide to shepherd you through a whole practice works really well for getting the most out of longer periods on your mat.

Don't be afraid to jot down a practice outline before you start. If it helps, you can take those notes and maybe even a watch with you onto your mat to help you keep track of time. With practice, you will find you need to do this less and less – especially any clock watching. But if it helps you meet your goal of practicing longer, then go for it!

How do I stay motivated to self-practice regularly?

We all want to listen to our bodies but also don't want to let the lazy sofa monster within us to keep us from doing anything productive. Finding the balance between these two is tricky! When is not practicing respectful of your body, and when is practicing the right decision?

The tool that will help the most here is Tool #12 What is Your Why? Finding the big driving reason behind why you want a yoga practice in your life – acknowledging it, writing it down, and writing down the smaller goals you are going to work towards to make it happen – is key. This will give you something to assess these tricky decisions against.

Spend some time on this tool. I know it is one of the easier ones to skip over but it will pay back every moment of time you commit to it.

I'm still stuck doing the same things over and over again in my self-practice. How do I get out of this rut?

Have an honest assessment of which of the tools you are using from this book and which ones you are not. Then try working your way through them ALL. Try new combinations and the different tips and tricks suggested in each one.

Tools #2 The Idea Generator, #3 Beats, #4 Breath, #5 Tuning In, #7 Change It Up and #8 Creative Flows are here specifically to help you inject something new into your practice, so focus on those first.

I also have more resources to help coming soon over at www.yoga-self-practice.com.

I don't feel like I'm progressing in my self-practice.

Having a teacher cheering us on to try something new or following an online video with lovely step-by-step instructions makes it A LOT easier to get out of our comfort zone.

But progressing in a self-practice can be so much more productive and efficient because you can take the exact amount of time necessary to work on all the elements you need to. Tools #16 to #20 are designed to help you here.

I don't work hard in my self-practice like I do when taking a class.

You need to challenge your thinking on this one. Yoga is not exercise, punishment, or simply about building muscles or fitness. It is about so much more than that. By merely starting a self-practice, you are already working HARD on your skills of self-discipline, perception, tuning in to yourself, finding comfort with discomfort, and accepting imperfection.

Maybe you don't get as sweaty, or try as many Chaturangas, especially if you are early in your self-practice journey. But you are pushing yourself in lots of other ways. You are working HARD. It's just a different type of work.

And if you do still crave those sweaty, crazy, feel-the-burn classes, then go and take them! Or you can use tools like #2 The Idea Generator, #3 Beats and #4 Breath to bring something new and fiery to your next self-practice.

I really hate practicing [insert your nemesis pose or category of poses here]. Should I be making myself do them in my self-practice?

There are two schools of thought on this one. The first says you should be leaning into what you are afraid of because that fear is telling you something about what you should be working on. The second says that making yourself do things you do not enjoy will become too high a hurdle and you just won't practice at all.

You need to decide for yourself on which end of this spectrum you sit. The answer may well be different for different poses/categories of poses.

For example, you might not practice handstands because of an old injury which will never resolve, but backbends you steer away from because you have never given them enough time to feel good.

If you are struggling to work this out, then go back to Tool #12. Finding your why for your practice will help you decide what is best FOR YOU.

I'm nowhere near doing all the fancy poses I see on Instagram and it's making me feel awful.

Unfollow. Unfollow. Unfollow.

Unfollow EVERYONE that makes you feel like this.

Yoga is for everyone: no matter their size, shape or ability. This is precisely why the community at @yogaselfpractice is committed to showing all this diversity.

We want YOU to be an active member of this community. Come over, ask questions, comment, share. We would love it to be the place you find YOUR yoga village (remember Tool #19).

I still don't really understand how to use all these tools!

20 tools. That is a lot of tools! Especially when you start combining them … There are over 2 million ways to do so. Eek!

Start small, start with what feels comfortable. Remember, 5 minutes is enough. YOU are enough.

I know you are meant to practice yoga in the morning, but I can't get up any earlier. What should I do?

You do not have to practice yoga in the morning for it to 'count'. If evenings work better for you, practice then. Maybe you can get away from your desk for a quick lunchtime practice. Great!

This is a practice that is meant to work FOR you. Ignore the 'rules': do what you can, when you can. THAT is yoga.

The Success Checklist

Last but not least, let's take a moment to celebrate your success: **big, small, and everything in between.**

It's easy to get caught up in the never-ending quest for MORE in yoga. More postures, more advanced versions, more time on your mat, more, more, more.

Check all that apply and add your own. Come back to this list when you are doubting yourself. There is also a blank version of this template in Part 8.

○ I have completed my first yoga self-practice

○ I feel more confident when it comes to my yoga practice

○ I have learned something new about my body as a result of independent time on my mat

○ I can see some of the mental benefits of practicing by myself

○ I am getting more comfortable with feeling awkward during my self-practice

○ I am getting better at listening to my body and understanding what it needs

○ I have been able to keep practicing even if I didn't get the flow identical on the 2nd side

○ I have tried different types of music, or no music at all, when I practice

○ I believe that any length or intensity of practice is enough

○ I have tried to learn something new and then given it a go in my own practice

○ I am getting more consistent in my self-practice

○ I am varying my practices depending on what I need on that given day

○ I have been able to see where I can tweak my asana after watching a video of it back

○ I have been kind to myself when I have struggled to get onto my mat for a yoga practice

○ I am starting to get an idea of which tools I can use in different circumstances

○ I manage to do either full or modified Savasana in most (or all!) of my self-practices

○ I am seeing physical progress is some of the postures in my practice repertoire

○ I am finding it less difficult to motivate myself to do a self-practice

○ I have tried five of the tools

○ I have tried ten of the tools

○ I have tried fifteen of the tools

○ I have tried all twenty tools!

"

If we practice yoga long enough, the practice changes to suit our needs. It's important to acknowledge that the practice isn't meant to be one practice for everybody.

The beautiful thing about yoga is that there are so many different approaches. As we go through our life cycles, hopefully we are able to find a practice that suits us.

And if you practice yoga long enough, that will change many times. What exactly that looks like is going to be different for each person

-

Tiffany Cruikshank

"

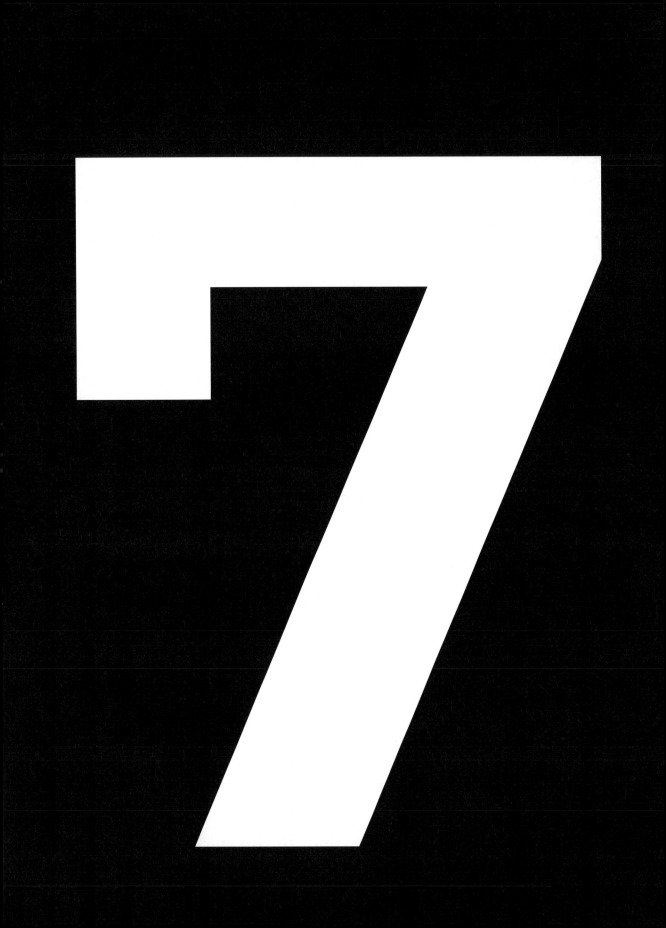

Glossaries & Further Reading

"

Constant practice alone
is the secret of success

-

Hatha Yoga Pradipika

"

Sanskrit: The Language of Yoga

Yoga is an ancient tradition originating from India: a traditional practice with indigenous roots.

To truly access the wisdom of the practice, we as practitioners must strive to honour this deep and wonderful history. Learning and using the classical language of Sanskrit is one of the many ways we can do that.

Prior to the early 1900s, the very way yoga survived was by a teacher speaking Sanskrit to a student. It was truly an oral tradition passed through the generations. The use of Sanskrit today pays homage to all that have come before us, connecting us to them and honouring them in a very real way.

Many of the Sanskrit names also have deeper meanings, which enlighten us further as to the original purpose of each posture and remind us that yoga is so much more than pure movement.

While The Pose Selector has both the English and the Sanskrit names for the postures, making the call to stick with the English names for postures in rest of the book was a decision I did not take lightly. Ultimately, I hope that readability and accessibility in a book written for those nearer the start of their yoga journey was the right call. However, this section is here to help you build your knowledge of this wonderful language and honour yoga's true Indian and Hindu roots.

Over the following pages, you will find two versions of a basic Asana Glossary. One sorted by the English words for the postures, and one sorted by the Sanskrit. Use these to expand your knowledge and to deepen your connection to the history and community of yoga through the ages.

Remember, you can download and/ or print blank copies of The Pose Selector template (and all the other templates in the book) at www. yoga-self-practice.com

English to Sanskrit Asana Glossary

Big Toe	Padangusthasana
Bird of Paradise	Svarga Dvidasana
Boat	Paripurna Navasana
Bound Angle	Baddha Konasana
Bound Extended Side Angle	Baddha Parsvakonasana
Bow	Dhanurasana
Bridge	Setu Bandha Sarvangasana
Camel	Ustrasana
Chair	Utkatasana
Child's	Balasana
Chinstand	Ganda Bherundasana
Cobra	Bhujangasana
Compass	Parivrtta Surya Yantrasana
Cow	Bitilasana
Cow Face	Gomukhasana
Crane	Kakasana
Crescent	Anjaneyasana
Crow	Bakasana
Dancer's	Natarajasana
Dolphin	Ardha Pincha Mayurasana
Downward-Facing Dog	Adho Mukha Svanasana
Eagle	Garudasana
Easy	Sukhasana
Eight-Angle	Astavakrasana
EPK 1	Eka Pada Koundinyanasana I
EPK 2	Eka Pada Koundinyanasana II

Extended Hand-to-Big-Toe	Utthita Hasta Padangustasana
Extended Side Angle	Utthita Parsvakonasana
Extended Triangle	Utthita Trikonasana
Fallen Angel	Devaduuta Panna Asana
Fire Log / Double Pigeon	Agnistambhasana
Firefly	Tittibhasana
Fish	Matsyasana
Flying Warrior	Visvamitrasana
Forearm Plank	Makara Adho Mukha Svanasana
Forearm Stand	Pincha Mayurasana
Forearm Wheel	Dwi Pada Viparita Dandasana
Gate	Parighasana
Goddess	Utkata Konasana
Half Bound Lotus Standing Forward Bend	Ardha Baddha Padmottanasana
Half Lord of the Fishes	Ardha Matsyendrasana
Half Moon	Ardha Chandrasana
Handstand	Adho Mukha Vrksasana
Happy Baby	Ananda Balasana
Head-to-Knee Forward Bend	Janu Sirsasana
Headstand	Sirsasana
Hero	Virasana
Heron	Krounchasana
High Lunge	Utthita Ashwa Sanchalanasan
Humble Warrior	Baddha Virabhadrasana
Intense Side Stretch	Parsvottanasana
King Pigeon	Kapotasana

English to Sanskrit Asana Glossary

Legs-Up-the-Wall	Viparita Karani
Locust	Salabhasana
Low Lunge	Anjaneyasana
Mountain	Tadasana
Noose	Pasasana
One-Legged King Pigeon	Eka Pada Rajakapotasana
One-Legged King Pigeon II	Eka Pada Rajakapotasana II
Peacock	Mayurasana
Pendant	Lolasana
Plank	Kumbhakasana
Plow	Halasana
Reclined Butterfly	Supta Baddha Konasana
Reclined Pigeon / Eye of the Needle	Supta Kapotasana
Reclined Twist	Supta Matsyendrasana
Reclining Hand-to-Big-Toe	Supta Padangusthasana
Reclining Hero	Supta Virasana
Reverse Plank	Purvottanasana
Revolved Head-to-Knee	Parivrtta Janu Sirsasana
Revolved Side Angle	Parivrtta Parsvakonasana
Revolved Triangle	Parivrtta Trikonasana
Sage's 1	Marichyasana I
Sage's 3	Marichyasana III
Scale	Tolasana
Seated Forward Bend	Paschimottanasana
Shoulder-Pressing	Bhujapidasana
Side Crane (Crow)	Parsva Bakasana

Side Lunge	Skandasana
Side Plank	Vasisthasana
Sphinx	Salamba Bhujangasana
Splits	Hanumanasana
Staff	Dandasana
Standing Forward Bend	Uttanasana
Standing Half Forward Bend	Ardha Uttanasana
Standing Split	Urdhva Prasarita Eka Padasana
Sugarcane	Chapasana
Super Soldier	Viparita Parivrtta Surya Yantrasana
Supported Shoulderstand	Salamba Sarvangasana
Tiger	Vyaghrasana
Tortoise	Kurmasana
Tree	Vrksasana
Upward Salute	Urdhva Hastasana
Upward-Facing Dog	Urdhva Mukha Svanasana
Warrior I	Virabhadrasana I
Warrior II	Virabhadrasana II
Warrior III	Virabhadrasana III
Wheel	Urdhva Dhanurasana
Wide-Angle Seated Forward Bend	Upavistha Konasana
Wide-Legged Forward Bend	Prasarita Padottanasana
Wild Thing	Camatkarasana
Yogi Push-Up	Chaturanga Dandasana
Yogi Squat	Malasana

Sanskrit to English Asana Glossary

Sanskrit	English
Adho Mukha Svanasana	Downward-Facing Dog
Adho Mukha Vrksasana	Handstand
Agnistambhasana	Fire Log / Double Pigeon
Ananda Balasana	Happy Baby
Anjaneyasana	Crescent
Anjaneyasana	Low Lunge
Ardha Baddha Padmottanasana	Half Bound Lotus Standing Forward Bend
Ardha Chandrasana	Half Moon
Ardha Matsyendrasana	Half Lord of the Fishes
Ardha Pincha Mayurasana	Dolphin
Ardha Uttanasana	Standing Half Forward Bend
Astavakrasana	Eight-Angle
Baddha Konasana	Bound Angle
Baddha Parsvakonasana	Bound Extended Side Angle
Baddha Virabhadrasana	Humble Warrior
Bakasana	Crow
Balasana	Child's
Bhujangasana	Cobra
Bhujapidasana	Shoulder-Pressing
Bitilasana	Cow
Camatkarasana	Wild Thing
Chapasana	Sugarcane
Chaturanga Dandasana	Yogi Push-Up
Dandasana	Staff
Devaduuta Panna Asana	Fallen Angel
Dhanurasana	Bow

Dwi Pada Viparita Dandasana	Forearm Wheel
Eka Pada Koundinyanasana I	EPK 1
Eka Pada Koundinyanasana II	EPK 2
Eka Pada Rajakapotasana	One-Legged King Pigeon
Eka Pada Rajakapotasana II	One-Legged King Pigeon II
Ganda Bherundasana	Chinstand
Garudasana	Eagle
Gomukhasana	Cow Face
Halasana	Plow
Hanumanasana	Splits
Janu Sirsasana	Head-to-Knee Forward Bend
Kakasana	Crane
Kapotasana	King Pigeon
Krounchasana	Heron
Kumbhakasana	Plank
Kurmasana	Tortoise
Lolasana	Pendant
Makara Adho Mukha Svanasan	Forearm Plank
Malasana	Yogi Squat
Marichyasana I	Sage's 1
Marichyasana III	Sage's 3
Matsyasana	Fish
Mayurasana	Peacock
Natarajasana	Dancer's
Padangusthasana	Big Toe
Parighasana	Gate

Sanskrit to English Asana Glossary

Paripurna Navasana	Boat
Parivrtta Janu Sirsasana	Revolved Head-to-Knee
Parivrtta Parsvakonasana	Revolved Side Angle
Parivrtta Surya Yantrasana	Compass
Parivrtta Trikonasana	Revolved Triangle
Parsva Bakasana	Side Crane (Crow)
Parsvottanasana	Intense Side Stretch
Pasasana	Noose
Paschimottanasana	Seated Forward Bend
Pincha Mayurasana	Forearm Stand
Prasarita Padottanasana	Wide-Legged Forward Bend
Purvottanasana	Reverse Plank
Salabhasana	Locust
Salamba Bhujangasana	Sphinx
Salamba Sarvangasana	Supported Shoulderstand
Setu Bandha Sarvangasana	Bridge
Sirsasana	Headstand
Skandasana	Side Lunge
Sukhasana	Easy
Supta Baddha Konasana	Reclined Butterfly
Supta Kapotasana	Reclined Pigeon / Eye of the Needle
Supta Matsyendrasana	Reclined Twist
Supta Padangusthasana	Reclining Hand-to-Big-Toe
Supta Virasana	Reclining Hero
Svarga Dvidasana	Bird of Paradise
Tadasana	Mountain

Tittibhasana	Firefly
Tolasana	Scale
Upavistha Konasana	Wide-Angle Seated Forward Bend
Urdhva Dhanurasana	Wheel
Urdhva Hastasana	Upward Salute
Urdhva Mukha Svanasana	Upward-Facing Dog
Urdhva Prasarita Eka Padasana	Standing Split
Ustrasana	Camel
Utkata Konasana	Goddess
Utkatasana	Chair
Uttanasana	Standing Forward Bend
Utthita Ashwa Sanchalanasan	High Lunge
Utthita Hasta Padangustasana	Extended Hand-to-Big-Toe
Utthita Parsvakonasana	Extended Side Angle
Utthita Trikonasana	Extended Triangle
Vasisthasana	Side Plank
Viparita Karani	Legs-Up-the-Wall
Viparita Parivrtta Surya Yantrasana	Super Soldier
Virabhadrasana I	Warrior I
Virabhadrasana II	Warrior II
Virabhadrasana III	Warrior III
Virasana	Hero
Visvamitrasana	Flying Warrior
Vrksasana	Tree
Vyaghrasana	Tiger

Further Reading

The possible further reading into yoga could take a lifetime. Below is a small selection of books that will hopefully be useful to those still in the early stages of that multi-year journey. They certainly helped me.

Anatomy & Postures

Tias Little | *Yoga of the Subtle Body: A Guide to the Physical and Energetic Anatomy of Yoga* (Shambhala Publications, Inc., 2016)
A practical guide to the anatomy of the physical, mental, emotional, and energetic body through the lens of yoga.

Leslie Kaminoff | *Yoga Anatomy* (Human Kinetics Europe Ltd, 2007)
An illustrated guide to postures, movements and breathing techniques.

Joanne Sarah Avison | Yoga: *Fascia, Anatomy & Movement* (Handspring Publishing, 2015)
A book that bridges the gap between application of traditional anatomy and real-life experiences of practicing (and teaching) yoga via a deep dive into fascia – the connective tissue that quite literally holds each of us together.

Donna Farhi | *Yoga Mind, Body & Spirit* (Henry Holt and Co., 2000)
This book centres around 75 fully illustrated asanas with descriptions of their executions and benefits. Farhi links these with the philosophical precepts of a yoga practice in a clear, concise style.

B.K.S Iyengar | *Light on Yoga: The Definitive Guide to Yoga Practice* (HarperThorsons, 2015)
A classic text for modern students of yoga. It contains a step-by-step photo-guide for different levels of practice, a guide to yoga breathing, and an introduction to the yoga philosophy.

Daniel Lacerda | *2100 Asanas: The Complete Yoga Poses* (Black Dog & Leventhal Publishers, 2015)
A photobook of 2100 different yoga postures.

General Yoga

Richard Freeman | *The Mirror of Yoga: Awakening the Intelligence of Body & Mind* (Shambhala Publications, Inc., 2010)
Richard Freeman presents an overview of the many teachings, practices, and scriptures that form the basis for all schools of yoga. He shows how the myriad forms are all related.

B.K.S Iyengar | *Light on Life: The Journey to Wholeness, Inner Peace, and Ultimate Freedom* (Rodale, 2005)
Iyengar walks us through the physical, emotional, mental, intellectual and spiritual elements of a yoga practice, showing why it is a way of living more than anything else.

William J. Broad | *The Science of Yoga: The Risks and the Rewards* (Simon and Schuster, 2012)
This book draws on more than 100 years of scientific research to provide an impartial answer on the benefits and potential costs of a modern-day yoga practice. Covering likelihood of injury, weight loss, mood enhancement, impact on fitness and much more. Essential reading!

Philosophy

Translation and Commentary by Sri Swami Satchidanandana | *The Yoga Sutras of Patanjali* (Integral Yoga Publications, 2012)
An in depth look at the Yoga Sutras, in Sanskrit, English and the meaning behind each.

Sadhguru | *Inner Engineering: A Yogi's Guide to Joy* (Penguin Random House India, 2016)
A clear and insightful guide to awakening your own inner wisdom, and one that makes that process an achievable practice. Accessible, light, and joyous. A must read.

Swami Vivekananda | *Raja Yoga: Conquering the Internal Nature* (Vedanta Pr, 1998)
Touching on different kinds of spiritual yoga – Bhakti, Karma – this book will walk you through your own will power and how to build true character, while you also learn about traditional Hindu stories.

"

As you go deeper into yourself, you will naturally come to realise that there is an aspect of your being that is always there and never changes. This is your sense of awareness, your consciousness.

It is this awareness that is aware of your thoughts, experiences the ebb and flow of your emotions, and receives your physical senses. This is the root of Self. You are not your thoughts; you are aware of your thoughts.

You are not your emotions; you are aware of your emotions. You are not your body; you look at it in the mirror and experience this world through its eyes and ears. You are the conscious being who is aware that you are aware of all these inner and outer things

-

Michael A. Singer

"

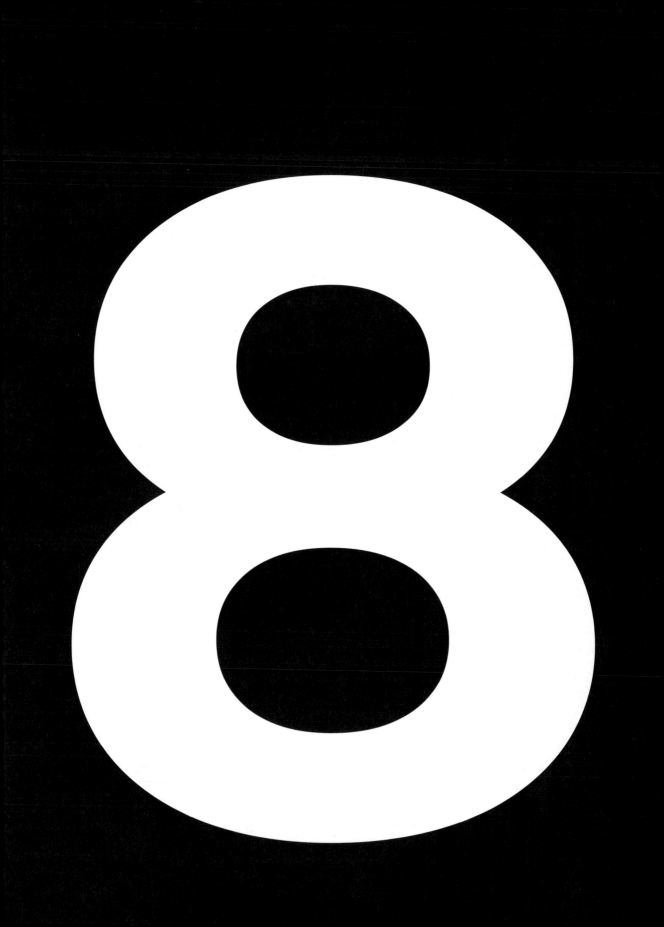

Templates

All of the following blank
templates are accessible to
download and/or print at
www.yoga-self-practice.com

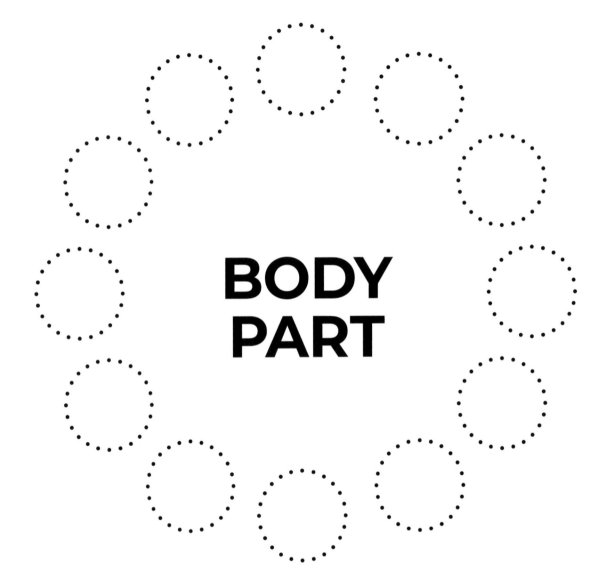

BODY
PART

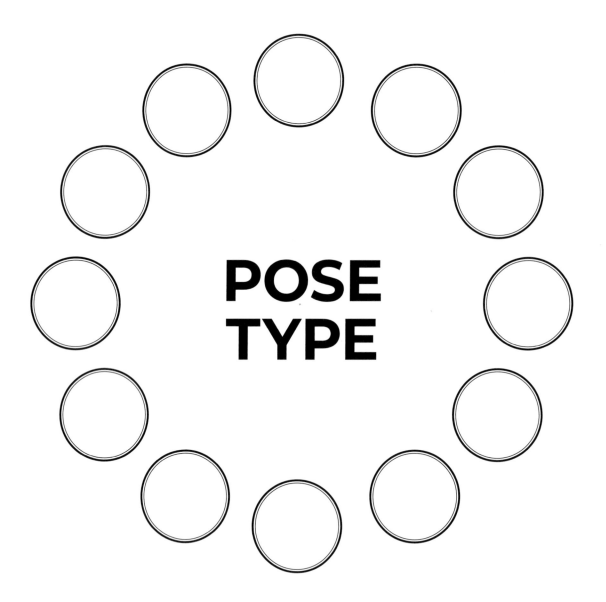

POSE
TYPE

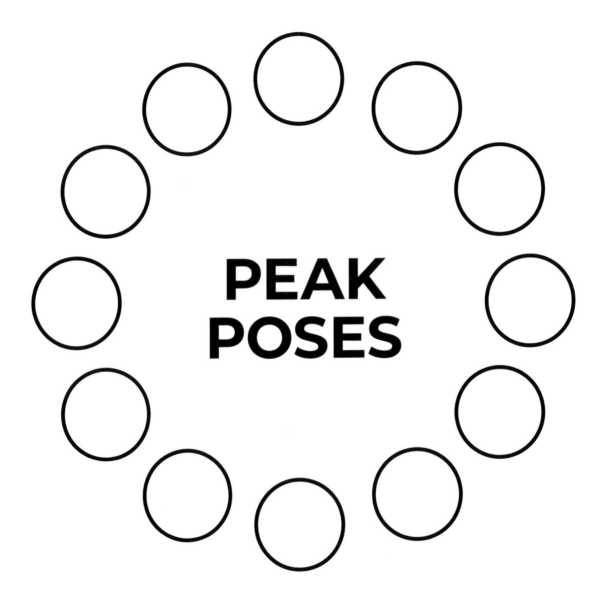

PEAK
POSES

Peak Pose	Pose Type	Body Part	

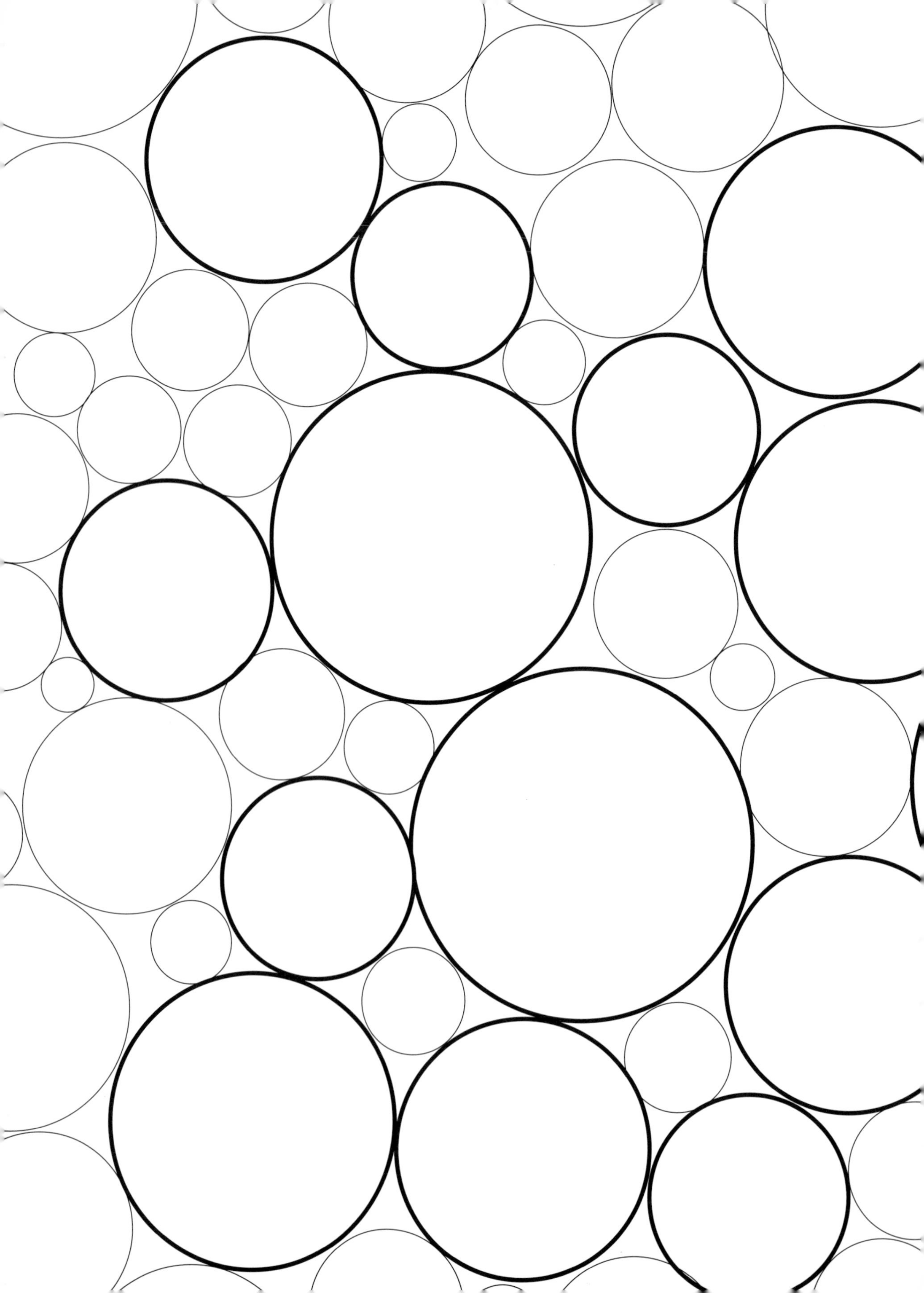

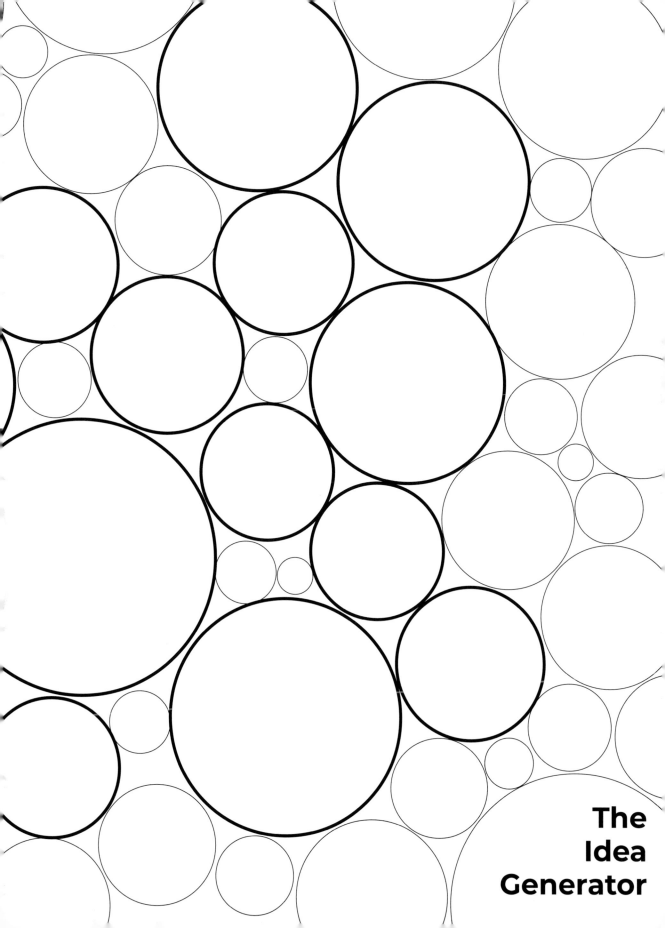

The
Idea
Generator

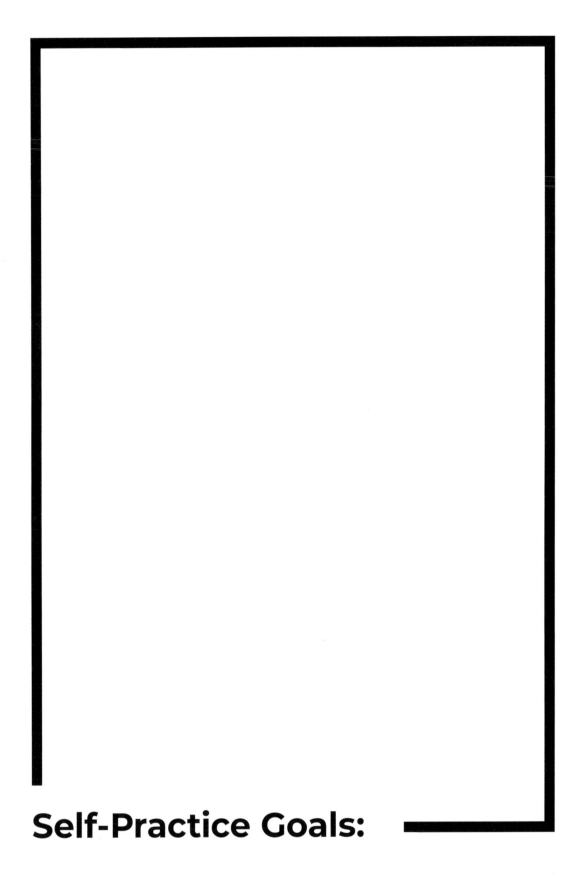

Self-Practice Goals:

A KISS Goals:

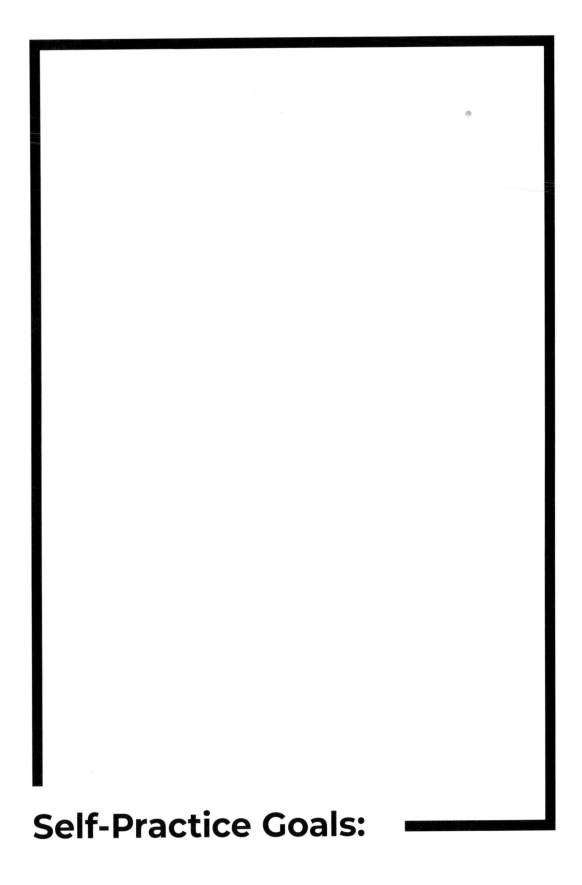

Self-Practice Goals:

A KISS Goals:

My Debrief Checklist	

What worked?

What didn't work?

How did it feel?

What was hard?

What came easy?

What might you do differently next time?

What surprised you the most?

My Debrief Checklist	

What worked?

What didn't work?

How did it feel?

What was hard?

What came easy?

What might you do differently next time?

What surprised you the most?

Weekly Journal Template	Self-Practice		Classes	
Monday				
Tuesday				
Wednesday				
Thursday				
Friday				
Saturday				
Sunday				
Time Spent: Total				

Weekly Journal Template	Self-Practice		Classes	
Monday				
Tuesday				
Wednesday				
Thursday				
Friday				
Saturday				
Sunday				
Time Spent: Total				

Weekly Journal Template	Self-Practice		Classes	
Monday				
Tuesday				
Wednesday				
Thursday				
Friday				
Saturday				
Sunday				
Time Spent: Total				

Weekly Journal Template	Self-Practice		Classes	
Monday				
Tuesday				
Wednesday				
Thursday				
Friday				
Saturday				
Sunday				
Time Spent: Total				

Practice Journal Template

Date:		Practice Info	

What I did:

How it felt:

Note to self:

Practice Journal Template

Date:		Practice Info	

What I did:

How it felt:

Note to self:

Yoga Prompt
Journal Template

Practice Info	

Favourite Pose(s) today:

Hardest Pose(s) today'

What worked, what didn't work:

What was hard, what came easy:

Something to do differently next time:

Something that surprised me in my practice:

Yoga Prompt
Journal Template

Practice Info	

Favourite Pose(s) today:

Hardest Pose(s) today'

What worked, what didn't work:

What was hard, what came easy:

Something to do differently next time:

Something that surprised me in my practice:

My Yoga Self-Practice Notes

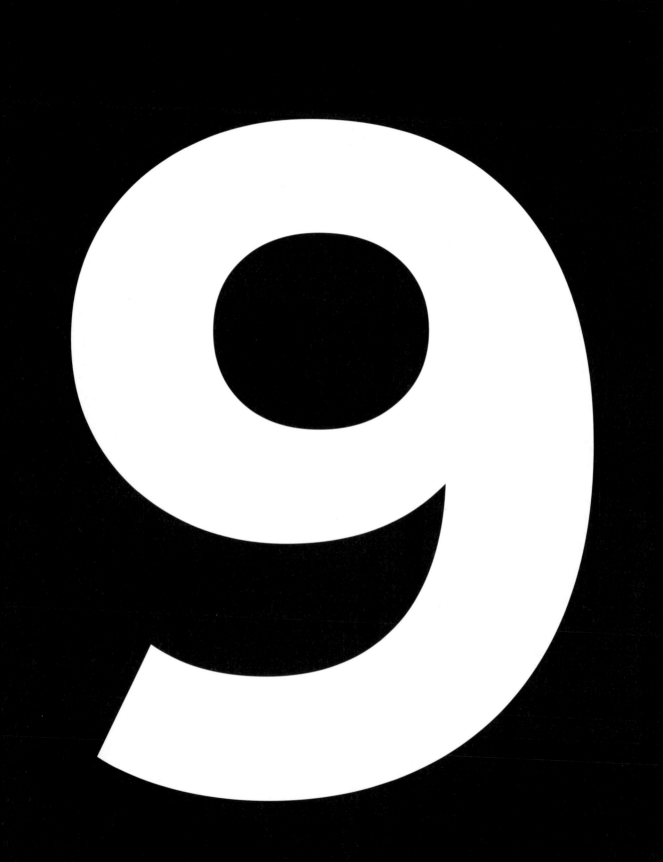

My Story & Acknowledgements

"

The success of
yoga does not lie
in the ability to
perform postures
but in how it
positively changes
the way we live
our life and our
relationships

-

T. K. S. Desikachar

"

My Story

What would become my yoga journey began quite literally with a bang when I was hit by a van while cycling to work through central London in the summer of 2015.

I was in my late twenties and had only been cycling for six months: the most 'sport' I had ever done in my life to date. I was NOT a girl who got picked to be on teams at school!

But after nine years of working long hours at a desk, I had been gently searching for something more active to introduce to my life. And the two-birds-with-one-stone element of cycle-commuting to work seemed to be that.

Even the broken collarbone and a badly damaged shoulder I sustained in the accident didn't stop me: I was back on my bike six weeks later.

However, some six months after that, I still could not lift my right arm above shoulder height, nor get it behind my back to do up my own bra. All despite having been to a few months of physiotherapy … (well, going to my once a week session and studiously doing absolutely none of the exercises I was given as homework).

Then in our last session, my physio suggested I try yoga. Specifically, Iyengar yoga: a type of yoga renowned for healing. It's characterised by long strong holds, slow deliberate movements and meticulous focus on alignment. Perfect for the injured, the not-so-young, and anyone brand new to yoga or physical movement.

So, I did.

And those first six or so months of just one or two classes a week were HARD. My broken body and jumpy mind couldn't manage any more yoga than that. My progress was achingly slow. Unwinding nearly 30 years of poor posture and ignorance of my body and its needs felt impossible at times.

But slowly things started to improve. I began to enjoy my time on the mat for its own sake rather than just looking to fix what was obviously broken.

As I gained basic strength and flexibility, I branched out, tried vinyasa yoga, and fell in love. More classes, more time, more patience, and a sprinkling of the magic of the yoga community via Instagram meant that by May 2017 I was doing my 200-hour yoga teacher training, all alongside working a very full-time job in the City of London as an Investment Banker.

For while I am truly passionate about yoga – about practicing it, teaching it, and sharing it – it is but one of my passions. I am passionate about my big career in finance. I am passionate about my husband. And I am passionate about the gorgeous son we recently brought into the world together.

I love living a life full of multiple passions. But when you have so many things you are passionate about, it is often rather challenging to fit them all into the 24 hours of a day.

As my career and my family grew, I found it harder and harder to carve out time to travel to and attend yoga classes. With so many other demands on my time, it was increasingly difficult to find the exact combination of yoga I wanted to practice on a certain day, be it in person or via online classes, from books or social media.

So I spent more and more time on my mat by myself.

5 minutes, 20 minutes, 90 minutes, 200 minutes and everything in between. Trying, failing, experimenting. Trying and failing again and again at being led by my body and my mind and my spirit on my mat.

I still went to as many classes as I could manage as I learn best from a teacher in real-life. And learning must always be a priority in the journey of yoga self-practice.

But the hours I spent on my mat alone (well, with my two cats as my Instagram will attest to!) were where I consolidated those learnings and where I learned even more about myself.

As I shared more of this on social media, the trickle of questions about how I learned to flow by myself turned into a torrent. I began to teach my yoga self-practice workshops in my home town of London. But there is only so much that can be squeezed into three hours.

Which led me here: an in-depth resource to help you start, develop and improve your own yoga self-practice. One that you can keep with you and use whenever you need it.

It is the guide I wish I had had with me. I only hope that the lessons it contains are as helpful to you as they have been to me.

Love

RAD xx

Acknowledgements

Nick

My editor-in-chief, my cheerleader, my sanity checker, my, well, my everything! Thank you for believing I could do this, even while juggling a career and a baby. Thank you for carving out the time and the space for me to do this, even when it meant shorter family walks or fewer miles on your bike or more evenings of me typing away not paying attention to you. We have always been sickeningly happy but these past few months of co-parenting and working on all of this together has taken that to places I could never have imagined. I love you more than you will ever know.

Simon

Designer extraordinaire. It has been a true privilege watching you bring this book to life, and I am in awe of your talent. I have always been proud to be your twin of course, but it has truly been a joy to work together on this.

You can see more of Simon's work and get in touch with him here: www.makeideasmatter.xyz | @agentbright777

Shahi

Editor, friend, yogi, professor, mum extraordinaire. If only California wasn't so far away.

Hannah

My sounding board on so many things life, and yoga, and motherhood. Thank you for listening to me talk at million miles an hour and always telling me that it was possible.

Adell and Celest

Your practices, friendships, passions and intellects have given me so much strength and even more inspiration. What else can I say apart from THANK YOU.

Chiara

My gifted illustrator. Thank you for turning my vision into reality on these pages.

You see can more of Chiara's beautiful work here: www.acupofcreativity.eu/

Happy self-practicing

self • practice

yoga

self • practice

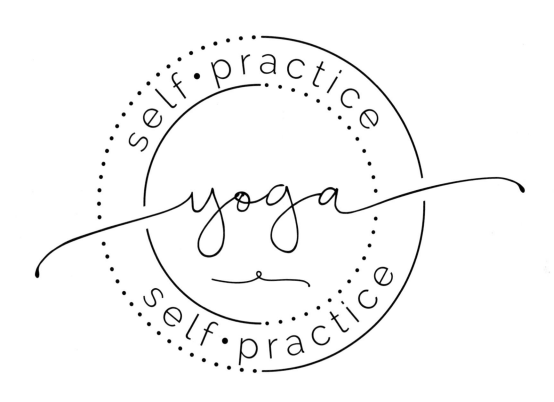